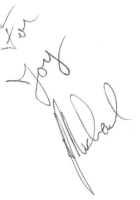

For
Joy

Michael

MW00618251

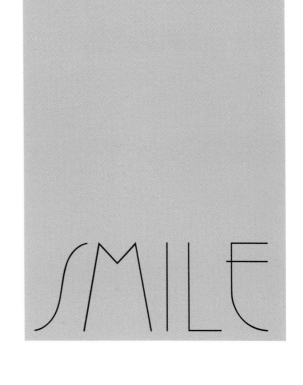

SMILE

How Dental Implants Can Transform Your Life

SMILE

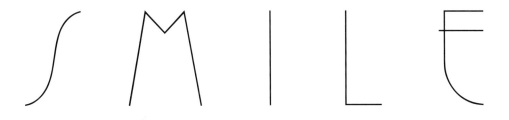

How Dental Implants
Can Transform Your Life

Michael R. Wiland, DDS
Michael Mastromarino, DDS
Joseph N. Pipolo

A KOERNER, KRONENFELD PUBLICATION

Published by

THE PARTHENON PUBLISHING GROUP
NEW YORK & LONDON

PUBLISHED IN ASSOCIATION WITH

Koerner, Kronenfeld Partners, LLC

112 Madison Avenue, 12th Floor

New York, New York 10016-744

by

The Parthenon Publishing Group Inc.

One Blue Hill Plaza

P.O. Box 1564

Pearl River, New York 10965

ISBN: 1-84214-082-5

Library of Congress Cataloging-in-Publication Data
Data available on request

Photo and Illustrations provided by Brånemark System®, Nobel Biocare USA, Inc.

Book and cover design by Lisa Vaughn, Two of Cups Design Studio, Inc.
Project management by Jane Lahr

Printed and bound by Butler & Tanner Ltd, Frome and London, UK

CONTENTS

WE WOULD LIKE TO DEDICATE THIS BOOK
TO THE FOLLOWING:

New York University

Mount Sinai Medical Center

Our wives and families

who stood by us and supported us through this process.

FOREWORD

Who is a candidate for this treatment? At one time, only a few short years ago—case selection was a sad process. Too many were refused treatment because of poor bone height, ridge width, nerve placement, and inappropriate sinus shapes. Today, for the most part, this is no longer the case. Bone grafting is a whole new ball game. Why? Because we can literally put bone wherever we need it, thereby reversing the ravages of time. Yet while we can accomplish this in one surgical session and initial healing takes only a week or so, the graft requires more time to integrate with the existing bone. Sometimes, it's true, implants can be placed simultaneously with the grafting process, other times graft healing requires its own healing period to become part of the patient's jaw.

The entire implant process is exciting for those of us who provide such care—especially those of us who studied dentistry before this "new age" of implantology matured to its present state of the art level. Every case we perform more than validates our present practice. Even so, implant dentistry is not for the patient (or the doctor) who demands instant gratification. Sure, we can schedule the surgery expeditiously and ask the lab to work overtime and compress our schedules, the one thing we cannot do is rush the biology of osseo-integration. Here we must be conservative and follow stated guidelines or else endanger the outcome. And with such astounding results, why risk failure? Implant case success rates fall in the high 90th percentile, a higher success rate than almost all other medical procedures. Even as I write, advances in genetically engineered proteins, bone growth factors, and new fixture designs are cutting the time between implant placement and final restoration. Undoubtedly, such advancements are just around the corner. Why, in the short period in which this book was written improved techniques have shortened the number of visits required for full restoration.

Quite frankly, if we have the full understanding, and the physical and financial cooperation of our patient, we can restore the jaws and mouth to look and function in ways that could not even be contemplated 25 years ago.

•8•   We created this book to provide potential patients with a full understanding of dental implants—the physical and financial cooperation is up to you.

We dedicate this book to the tens of thousands of patients who trusted a new technology and are now enjoying implant-supported teeth, because you are the most important part of the team that makes this treatment work.

We would like to categorically state that there is nothing like your own teeth, and the dentist's primary responsibility is to repair and preserve them. However, when these original teeth fail they can be replaced, in many instances, not only with removable dentures or crown and bridge dentistry, but with root form implants and a variety of replacements which allow patients to function normally.

As a species we are living longer. At the turn of the century the average life span was 50 years; at present we are living into our late 80s, nor is relative good health uncommon at 90. The International Longevity Center US predicts that life spans of 120 will no longer be out of the ordinary in another quarter century. That's the good news. The bad news is that various body parts wear out. The logical solution to this problem being replacement. Just as orthopedists replace hips, knees, shoulders, etc.—dentists replace teeth with implants.

Scientists predict that we will soon be living 30 % longer, the question which follows is: What quality of life can the "new" elderly expect? If we eat nutritious foods, can chew and fully digest them, we stand a better chance of living to a happy, healthy and vital advanced age. Dental implants allow people to enjoy all foods, a laugh-out-loud and full robust SMILE. The rest is up to you.

Introduction

How to Use this Book

The subject of dental implants is never going to compete with a Stephen King novel as a page turner. You won't see too many copies of this book packed along with suntan lotion and taken to the beach. Dentists and surgeons are going to prefer the technical language of some of our source books, and people without need of implants (or whose loved ones aren't in need of implants) will not be drawn to this material for "recreational reading." Buyers of this book, therefore, will read about the two-stage surgery common to 98% of successful implants, and then proceed directly to the chapter which refers to their specific condition.

One question which kept recurring during the writing of this book was: How technical should we get? One member of the team thought we shouldn't be technical at all, another thought details were important. Not surprisingly, we ended up compromising. In our visit-by-visit approach, those of you who seek general information will find "the bottom line," at the top, labeled "In Short," while the technically minded are invited to read on for an "In Depth" discussion. Sections entitled "Meanwhile, back at the Lab…" will likewise explain certain behind-the-scenes technologies crucial to making implants a rock-hard reality.

• | | •

If you are a natural-born student who, once interested in a subject, is inspired to learn it "bottom to top," then—please—read us front to back. Yet in this increasingly busy world it is more likely that you will want to know, immediately, ARE DENTAL IMPLANTS FOR ME? And if so, HOW MUCH WILL THEY COST? and HOW MUCH WILL THEY HURT? and HOW LONG WILL IT TAKE? and HOW LONG WILL THEY LAST? This is why we've designed this book with a general introduction to the subject (the super-busy can skip the history), followed by the step-by-step examination of the two-stage surgeries central to all state-of-the-art implants. From here we branch off into specific cases—a majority of readers will "bone up" on the procedure which directly concerns them.

We've again used our brief "bottom line" breakdown to review the basics while modifying certain information specific to each different type of implant, while continuing to mark "in-depth" discussions as before.

Finally, we conclude each procedural chapter with an interview with a patient who has been through exactly what was described. In this way, you get to hear the ups and downs of the implant procedure.

Big Words...

We have also struck something of a compromise between lay language and technical terminology. Technical jargon, if understood, provides a far more precise understanding of any field it describes. For the general reader, however, such language creates a minefield through which some become reluctant, even fearful, to proceed. The term "X-ray" for instance, is understood by a general readership. "Panorex X-ray," while more accurate, may frustrate easy understanding. This is why we've simplified many terms, sacrificing a more complete mastery, in favor of general comprehension. When we do use more difficult terms they will appear in parentheses, following a simple explanation. The explanation, and the "big word," therefore, appear side-by-side. This is why we hope the glossary in the back will not be as necessary to your understanding as it would be in a text on the subject.

Sorry, No Blood...

• 13•

Again, for you Stephen King fans out there, we apologize. Although virtually all first-and-second stage implant surgeries do, of course, involve that bodily fluid so valued by vampires— we have chosen to underplay this aspect of our specialty. While we do not deny it, we do not revel in it. Anyone wishing to see actual photographs of implant surgeries, we hereby direct you to our bibliography. Also, for those of you who have noted that the best dentists are failed comedians compulsively telling jokes to an audience not only captive, but in most cases, gagged, we extend no apology whatsoever.

CHAPTER ONE

The Basics of

DENTAL

Implants

Why Are You Here?

Nobody walks into a dentist's office for fun. You walk in because you have a problem involving pain, inability to eat, vanity, or all of the above. And if you're considering a dental implant, chances are you don't have a little problem—more likely you've got a big one.

Put your feet up, take a breath, relax. You've come to the right place. First, we're going to sit down and talk about human teeth in general, so you can get a better idea as to why you've reached this point of asking about dental implants. Then we'll tell you a little about this revolutionary movement in dentistry involving implants and its history. Primarily, however, we'll use the majority of this book to talk about you, and how you can be helped with dental implants.

About Your Mouth: The Possibility of Dentures

A healthy adult has a mouth filled with 32 permanent teeth. We are equipped with a smaller set of teeth as children. Look on those as a practice set, as the training wheels on which some of us learn basic dental hygiene. Elephants, which live 80 years and beyond, feature three sets of teeth. When the third set goes, so does the elephant. Inability to chew is a death sentence for a mammal. This is also true of primitive human cultures, though at our present level of medical sophistication, we have doubled life expectancy even though we still only have only two sets of natural teeth.

Because the Homo sapiens body evolved to serve an average life span of roughly half a century, our teeth, like hundreds of other features of human anatomy, break down as we age. Good dental hygiene helps, but only to a point. Health practitioners and advocates aren't immortal either. Even Jack La Lanne will one day die.

All that lives must eat, and to eat, all mammals, including humans, must chew. If an average American chews a million times every three years, a 75-year-old woman will have chewed 25 million times, mostly on her second set of teeth. Could she chew another two or three million times on the same old teeth? Possibly. What if she lives to be 95 and clocks in another 20 million chomps?

In this latter extreme case, it becomes physically impossible to maintain the original equipment. Ditto the experience of most modern adults whose diets vary with shows on the food channel, new restaurants, or the latest in splashy junk-food advertising campaigns. The combined pressure of the jaws places thousands of pounds of pressure per square inch on our primary chewing areas; tooth make-up simply cannot withstand such punishment. No matter how well maintained, a 95-year-old's teeth cannot go the distance. And neither can most "healthy" sets of teeth, given what we put them through these days.

In our files we have several patients of 95 who have had dental implants for ten years already—ten years of active life! The fact of the matter is there will be more and more 95-year-old people who will need more and more artificial teeth. To a majority of educated Americans, this still means dentures.

If you believe the advertisements for the glue that holds a pair dentures on the naked gum, then false teeth aren't so bad. But if you remember rushing to give grandmother a good-morning kiss only to find her teeth in a jar—you know better. Dentures are like wigs, they start at mediocre and only get worse. Truthfully, eating an apple with dentures is about as likely as finding a politician without a skeleton in the closet.

Beyond The Past: The Revolution in Dentistry

For centuries, doctors of dentistry have sought to repair and replicate human anatomy to the best of their abilities. False teeth were often animal teeth carved down to fit into the holes left by the work of a pair of pliers wielded by barbers, tinkers, traveling actors—anyone with courage enough to be ruthless. Indeed, dentists of the past inspired fear and loathing of a type which is today saved exclusively for lawyers.

What's changing the way we think about dentistry? For one thing, at the top of the profession we're better than good; we're in fact good enough to build a business based on trust. The spooky sadist in the mask is gradually transforming into an angel of mercy who has given you back dining, dating, and laughing out loud. Furthermore, properly maintained implants last longer than "original parts." And if—against the odds—an implant is damaged, repair usually amounts to little more than a single visit to your restorative dentist.

Implants harken to a veritable fountain of youth—at least as far as eating and socializing go. Today's dentist can restore your face, your smile, and with it—a fair share of self esteem.

NATURE'S GIFT: THE SMILE

While maintaining pain-free and disease-free teeth is dentistry's first function, its second function—and nearly as important— is the overall care for the instinctive "showing-of-teeth," that single-most important communication in life commonly known as the smile.

From the day we become aware of a smiling, protective parent, through the days when we smile in friendship to those beyond our families, to the day we smile in such a way as to create families of our own—glistening teeth speak of a joy in the presence of others: a visual, nonverbal signature unique to each and every individual.

When a smile is damaged, so too is the effect that that smile has upon the world, and the effect that the world has upon the smile. Most people afflicted with broken, stained or rotting teeth soon learn to cover their mouths as their dental hygiene deteriorates. And they tend to smile less and less frequently until they hardly smile at all.

This is why restoring a smile also tends to restore a person's reasons to smile. The maintenance of a smile speaks volumes about how worthwhile a person feels about him or herself. How many smile-afflicted persons find romance has fallen out of their lives completely? How many find themselves eating mushy, overcooked food by themselves and hiding their teeth behind hands in a contrived manner? All right, it's not the end of the world. It's just a gradual lessening, a diminishment, part of the larger attrition of pleasure in daily life which it is our job as health workers to correct. And we can.

Ever notice how those who afford themselves the unabashed privilege of a smile seem to get more out of life? Or how an unconstricted smile need not be picture perfect in order to act as a magnifier of joy? The reason being that a smile is—ninety-nine times out of a hundred—an enjoyable sight. As one 1960's balladeer notably observed: "When you smile at me I will understand, for that is something everybody everywhere does in the same language."

How We Started

Speaking for ourselves, when we first formed our implant dentistry team we made the mistake of placing a large advertisement in the Yellow Pages announcing a cooperative clinic of dentists and technicians specializing in dental implants. Response was heavy but so completely misinformed that it soon became necessary for our receptionists to spend extensive periods of time on the phones re-educating one confused person at a time, very few of whom committed to treatment. The upshot? We discontinued the ad. Yet it was those frustrating, seemingly wasted hours that initiated the education process which resulted in this book.

We're going to assume that—like those Yellow Pages readers first calling our office—you, or someone near to you, is considering a dental implant procedure. We're also going to assume you've heard all sorts of good and bad reports about all sorts of different kinds of implants, and that you are in search of an accurate accounting.

So What is a Dental Implant... And Will it Hurt?

A dental implant is a bionic replacement; a tooth-replica anchored in your jawbone. Since it is not a tooth, however, it has no nerves, and therefore can feel no pain. It is totally artificial, completely unnatural, and even if it functions beautifully and looks very natural, indeed, it is a total fabrication. And that's good news.

For while teeth and gums abound with nerves, the jaws have very few—thus there are less pain sensors in implantology than in conventional dentistry. Proper implant procedures take time, but statistically result in less pain than crown and bridge dentistry or even many "simple" fillings. Furthermore, properly maintained implants last longer than "original parts," and if—while unlikely—an implant is damaged, repair usually amounts to little more than undoing a screw—removing, repairing, restoring the implant—and screwing it back into place again. Natural teeth are complex things. They're essentially living organs that, like most parts of the body, come connected to the rest of what keeps you living. They're made up of a root, a crown and a pulp organ, all hooked into one's jawbones with gum tissue and a nerve system that's been put in place, like an alarm system, to let you know when things are going wrong. Unfortunately, as with most parts of one's body, things can go wrong with one's teeth. They decay. They become unhinged from the jawbone. They fall out, or need to be removed. They stop working.

• 22 • An implant is a metal facsimile of a tooth with porcelain coating designed to look like the real thing. Its key component is a titanium anchor that melds into the jawbone. These are made of titanium because this special element has been found to be the only non-corrosible metal that the body will not reject; it is bio-inert, and thus totally compatible with the human body. Before the titanium anchor (technically: a fixture fitted with an abutment) is loaded with the porcelain-coated tooth (prosthesis), it has become part of your jawbone. That's why several months elapse between the first procedure and the last.

"Fixtures" and "abutments" are not dental implants. Nor are the "prostheses" (replacement teeth) dental implants. A dental implant is both of these components, with several other pieces of hardware joined to them. To "dentally implant" is also a verb. It is a thing we do while employing an entire workshop of tools with new duties to help us perform new techniques to recreate the appearance and function of young, strong, healthy teeth.

When an implant is complete, then, it functions like a tooth as regards chewing and smiling, but not in terms of feeling or decay.

What's The Story?
A Brief History of Implants

The first recorded instance of dental implantology was a copper spike hammered into the upper jaw of an Egyptian king some 3,000 years ago. But this work was probably done by the undertaker to improve his smile in the underworld. The first evidence of such an operation upon the living had to wait another thousand years and was accomplished in what is now Honduras. Similar surgeries included replacing lost human teeth with those of dogs, goats, and monkeys. Other teeth were obtained from slaves and the poor, who parted with their chompers for a price, after which wealthy patrons evidently tolerated dental "replanting" sessions. Subsequent cultures found the elite too pain-sensitive for such procedures, thus the further history of implants awaited the age of anesthesia. What hangs between is the history of fake teeth, the competitive brother to implants, which dominated the scene for thousands of years. We read of these in the Talmud when a young woman procures a fake tooth to please her fiancé; and in Roman law, which forbade the funeral burial of jewelry until an amendment passed in 450 B.C. allowed for corpses to be interred with gold contrivances

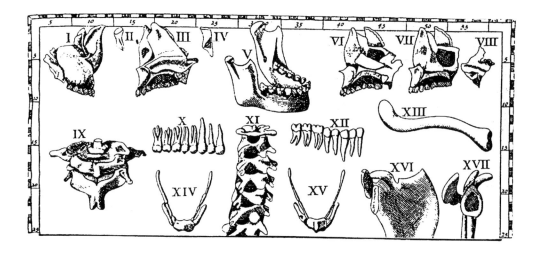

Accurate renderings of the entire mouth were first created by the roman anatomist, Eustachius, who also first identified the tube between the ear and throat bearing his name. Eustachius' *Libelus de Dentibus* ("Pamphlet on the Teeth") remained the definitive work on the subject until the 18th century. These engravings of canine, premolar, molar, upper and lower incisors, although created in 1552, were not published until 1714, due more than likely, to the secrecy surrounding such surgical knowledge.

holding in false teeth. The Roman satirist Martial (who died circa 103 A.D.) provides us with socio-sexual awareness of dental hygiene:

Lucania has white teeth, Thais brown. How comes it?
One has false teeth, one her own.
And you, Galla, lay aside your teeth at night
Just as you do your silken dress.

A great deal of barbaric guesswork as practiced by barbers, surgeons, doctors was finally consolidated into the first real textbook of dentistry by Pierrre Fauchard [p 161] in his "Treatise on the Teeth," in 1728. Previous contributions are attributable to the anatomist Vesalius (1514-1564), his student, Eustachius

(?- 1574) and the gradual improvement of surgical practices in general. Throughout the Middle Ages, the faithful would simply pray to St. Apollonia, patron saint of dentists, in hopes that their pain would be divinely lifted—or the usually brutal dentist would have his ruthless hand angelically guided.

In the New World, colonist ingenuity did not linger long behind European sophistication, Boston fast became a city famous for advancements in dentistry. In the rear pages of the "Boston Gazette," September 19, 1768, soon-to-be-Americans read:

PAUL REVERE
All persons who have had false teeth loosen (as they will in Time) may have them fastened by the above.

•25•

Twenty years and a revolution later George Washington, in a letter to one of his dentists, complained that his dentures "are

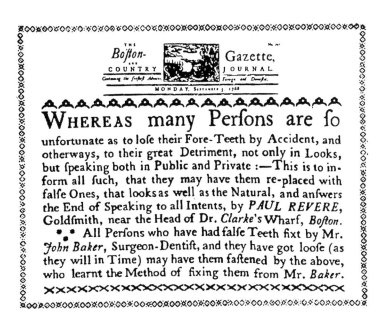

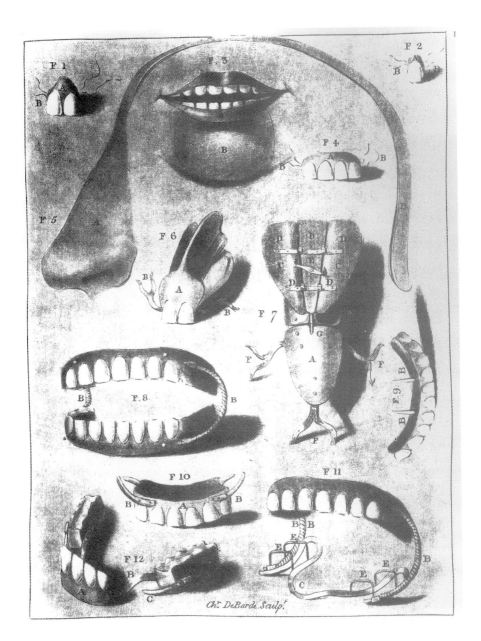

A page from "Dissertation on Artificial Teeth" (1997) shows de Chemant's arsenal of prosthetics—some of the first porcelain teeth ever made—as well as an artificial nose, a disfigurement caused by the as-yet incurable syphilis.

uneasy in the mouth." Though the father of our country had many sets of dentures, none of them were made of wood (as legend insists). His favorite set, created by a certain John Greenwood, consisted of human teeth set in an ivory base. These clappers were hinged with a spring, which gave Washington considerable trouble while talking and eating.

It was another Frenchman, Alexis Duchateau, who invented the porcelain denture, and another, Nicolas Dubois de Chemant, who perfected, popularized, and imported these (along with their inventor) to English high society while its Parisian counterparts were having their heads cut off in the French Revolution. However, the invention of individual porcelain teeth, which again revolutionized denture designs in the early 1800s, is credited to the Italian dentist Giuseppangelo Fonzi.

•27•

In 1800 the American dentist James Gardette accidentally discovered that suction alone could hold dentures to the naked gums, thereby dispensing with the wires, springs, and loops of early dentures. Two-piece affairs appeared, made of gold, porcelain, platinum, and lead—the last of which we today know to be poisonous.

In 1839 another savvy American by the name of Charles Goodyear discovered that adding sulfur to rubber hardened it most usefully. His son, Charles Jr., used this "vulcanized" rubber to create dentures which dominated the market until the 1930s, when plastics appeared.

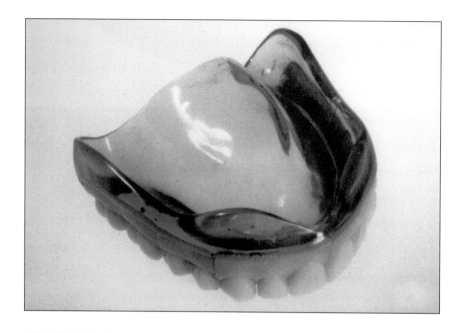

The futuristic look of celluloid seen here in this upper denture, circa 1880, in fact, did not seriously threaten the preeminence of vulcanized rubber. The celluloid stained easily, absorbed odors and proved flammable.

Then, in 1939, approximately 3,000 years after the first copper stud was nailed into an Egyptian's mouth, implantology awoke from its cosmic nap when two dentist brothers from Boston, by the name of Stock, screwed a false tooth in place and X-rayed the results. This bold operation anticipated the Italian, Formiggini's "cork screw" implant of 1940, which most histories credit as the first instance of dental implants in modern times. Chercheve soon introduced a further screw-type post made of chrome cobalt. In 1966 Leonard Linkow invented and popularized "blade" implants, which he hammered into the jawbones of thousands of patients. He claimed a success rate of 91%, while independent research found five-year success rates between 42% and 66%.

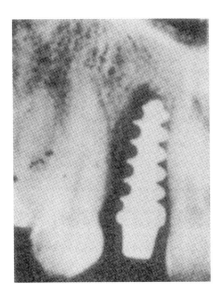
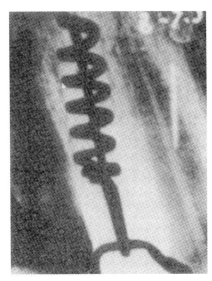

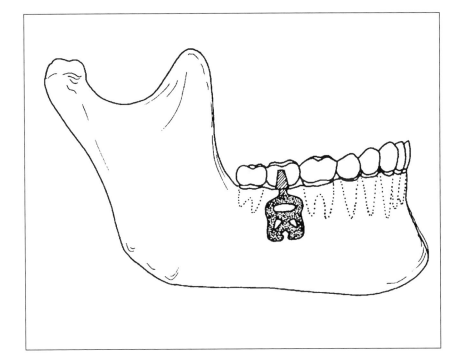

Top: Dental implants' early efforts: a solid screw by Stock Brothers of Boston, 1939; and a corkscrew by Formiggini in the 1940s. Bottom: Lower jaw with blade implant popularized by Dr. Leonard Linkow.

In 1967 Hodosh, attempting a return to the ancient "adopt-a-tooth" style of implant, placed acrylic fully rooted teeth into the jaws of baboons. These and all subsequent human implants, his research claims, met with full acceptance into bone tissue. Other independent researchers could not duplicate his experiments or his successes.

Other "nouvelle" techniques were developed, such as the construction of a wire saddle supporting implants which straddled the jawbone without actually piercing bone (subperiosteal implants). Another method drilled clear through the jawbone and placed implants screwed into a metal plate on the other side of the lower jaw. There were tripodal implants, Ramus struts, zygomatic implants—the list goes on.

•30•

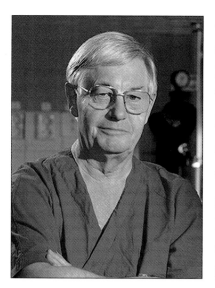

A good ten years before Linkow and Hodosh, however, Dr. Per-Ingvar Brånemark, Professor of The Institute for Applied Biotechnology at the University of Goteborg, Sweden, discovered the most important principle of modern Dental Implantology. While working with bone repair mechanisms, he observed and coined the term "osseointegration." This was the process by which a titanium chamber surgically inserted into the tibia of a rabbit was accepted by the specimen without infection. Other substances, including several already mentioned, didn't test with anywhere near the results of titanium. As early as 1952, then, the Branemark system was perfecting hip replacement procedures.

It wasn't until the mid-60s, however, that Brånemark turned his attention to the field of dentistry, placing titanium mounts into the jaw bones of dogs, onto which infection-free prosthetic teeth were soon attached. By 1971, Brånemark perfected standardized surgical components and drilling equipment which, together with his streamlined methodology, introduced an entirely new science to dentistry. While more than 30 other systems subsequent to Brånemark's now flood the market, with a 96.5% success rate after five years, and 86% success rate after 15 years, (as well the complete satisfaction of the very first implant patient of 35 years ago), the Swedish original is acknowledged as the gold standard of implantology.

Where We Are Today:
The Brånemark Breakthrough

Having clinically observed implant case studies for over 20 years it is safe to say that the results of Brånemark treatments are both successful and predictable. The Swedish system established a precedent for all subsequent dental implant work by introducing two separate procedures. First titanium anchors are set in bone by a surgeon. Then, after 90-120 days of healing, the surgeon exposes the implant and attaches a healing cap onto the bone-fast foundation. Ten days later, the restorative dentist takes over, and, in conjunction with the lab staff, essentially constructs a work of functional sculpture in your mouth; one that will defy the ravages of time and the propensity to decay.

The six components comprising a single tooth implant, in the Brånemark system, represent the first successful dental refabrication which does not depend on any pre-existing teeth. Underlying bone, and bone alone, supports the free-standing replacement. Since this replica is stronger than its human companions, properly maintained implants (similar to mechanical hips and knees) will tend to outlast the mortal body they serve. Today, state-of-the-art dental implantology development has spurred the growth and development of bone grafting techniques which have raised the science to new standards. Injuries and deteriorations, which ten years ago were considered untreatable, are currently meeting with truly miraculous results. We will take a closer look at bone grafting in a future chapter.

First we need to know more about you.

Tell Us About Yourself: Personal Questions Involved in Implants

Any implant procedure requires a clinical examination. Just as with any implant, dental implants must be customized to your mouth and dental needs.

We will take panorex X-rays of your upper and lower jaws. Your medical history will be reviewed carefully. It's not that we work

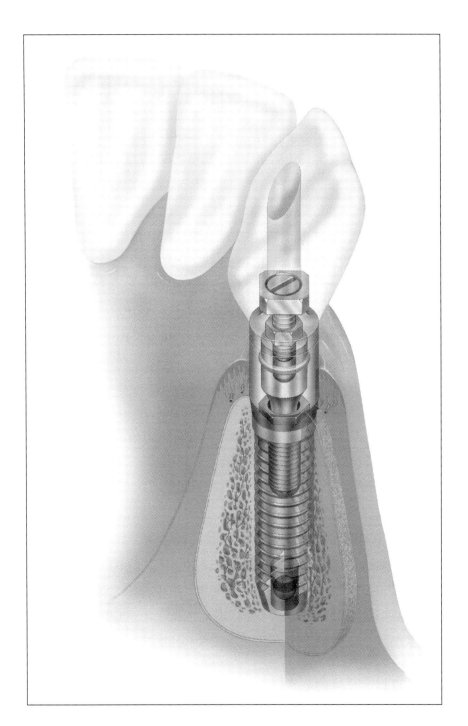

This is a complete dental implant ready to function.

with the FBI—it's that such information is necessary to make you orally functional and whole again.

Once you sit in the chair, open your mouth and go, "ahhh," we quickly ascertain the state of your gums, jaws, and teeth. If you suffer from gingivitis or other gum diseases, we will rate you as either hopeless, poor, compromised, fair, or good—but even the worse case of periodontal disease need not prevent successful implants, if you work with us! We will check your bite and mobility of teeth, whether they meet properly—how much they rock. Gradually, we will ascertain the geography of your mouth, including not only the teeth but the jawbone from which they grow.

• 34 • With today's radiographs and CAT scans we will know exactly the shape of your sinuses, and the levels and density of the bone which delineates the sinus-bottom. We will know how deep your gums are, how strong they are, and how strong the bone is upon which they sit.

The fact is that, because an implant is fastened directly to your jaw, bone is our first concern—assuming you're otherwise healthy. It turns out that without a proper foundation, Brånemark's technologies (and all the other implant systems based on his) are useless. As in the building of a house, the very first concern is foundation. Take young children for instance; while bone is indeed strong enough to support implants, facial growth will change the configuration of bone structure such that the "groundwork" will fundamentally change. For this reason children are not acceptable candidates for most implants.

On the other hand, an implant placed in the mouth of a young adult accident victim is ideal.

It is often (improperly!) thought that older patients or ones suffering from gum disease will need bone grafting before successful implant surgery can take place. This is one of the most often repeated misconceptions in dentistry. It is not age which is the criteria, but fitness. When teeth—even old teeth—are used, the gums and the bone upon which the gums sit remain vital. When teeth are pulled and dentures replace them, the gums retract and the bone resorbs (shrinks), this is an atrophying (stagnating or devitalizing) process which is not reversed by implants. This is why it's important to hold onto your natural teeth unless their removal is necessary to the greater good of your mouth.

We have seen cases of people in their 40s with far worse bone atrophy than people in their 80s. Why? Loss of teeth early and the resultant resorption of bone. This isn't to say that old people who have been wearing dentures for 20 years won't have bone loss, they will. But age is not the issue.

In some borderline cases "spot" grafting can accompany the placement of abutments; other times we must add bone with a preliminary procedure which has its own recuperation period prior to the formal implant process. We will go into this in more depth in a subsequent chapter devoted exclusively to the subject.

Natural is Better, Painless is Best:
When to Get an Implant

Dentists don't have to invent problems to make a living. In our office (and in all responsible dental facilities) we do everything practically possible to preserve existing teeth. Proud as we are of the remarkable strides implantology has taken and is taking, we are just as proud to "shore up" a still functioning mouth. Why? Because given a choice, natural teeth are always better. It's that simple. Unfortunately, there sometimes comes a moment in age or in illness when "fixing the old" becomes more frustrating, painful, and expensive than "ushering in the new." Recognizing this point of diminishing returns is crucial to proper implantology; a good dentist passes on a fair share of bad news concerning doomed teeth and the like. The good news is that comfortable and affordable implants can end the pain and embarrassment once and for all.

However, if you are not comfortable with your dentist's advice, maybe you have the wrong dentist. Trust is a huge issue in all health care, but since so much pain and fear are associated with dentistry, it is doubly important that we believe in the competence, fairness, and perhaps even in the humanity of our dentist. This is part of the reason modern dentists find themselves describing their profession as "the business of trust."

Many patients, especially the elderly, while generous with children and grandchildren, can become parsimonious when it comes to their own wants and needs. Investing in your mouth is a huge statement of self-worth. Some people, like the lady you are about to read about, must be pushed into dental implants. Years down the line they are extremely grateful for the coercion.

Again, it's a question of trust.

The basic responsibility of your dentist is to keep your teeth working painlessly and attractively. Just how to best accomplish this must vary in accordance with budget, health, attitude, and the 1,001 differences that make us each unique.

A trumpeter needs a mouth with a strong foundation through which to blow into a mouthpiece. The higher the note, the harder the mouthpiece is pressed against the teeth and gums. If a denture moves—a solo is ruined. A 15-year-old has had braces put on too early and too tight, his/her teeth fall out. A top model is in a motorcycle crash with her rock-star boyfriend. Her "signature" smile is wrecked, and needs to be rebuilt. With the Lloyds' of London insurance money, price is no object. Could these people be candidates for dental implants? Absolutely. What about disease victims? Those born with a cleft palate or other oral birth defect, or those who for reasons of age, illness, or injury are missing all their natural teeth in one or both jaws? Yes, yes, yes—all could be candidates for dental implants. But how many, which kind, where, and for how long a recovery, and how much will it cost?

These are some of the reasons dental implants vary to suit the needs and means of the patient.

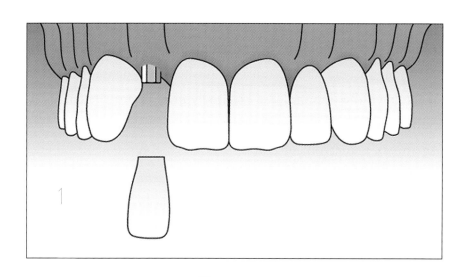

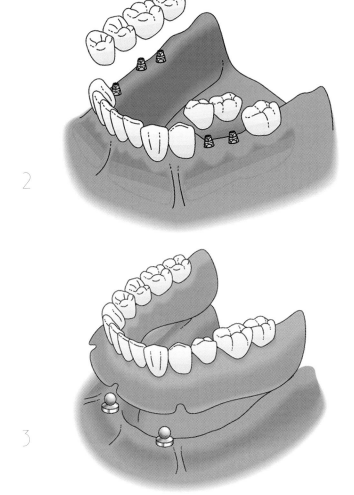

THE THREE SHAPES AND THREE TYPES OF IMPLANTS . . .

The first difference is that implant restorations come in three basic configurations: single tooth, partial arch, and entire arch. [See figure] A second difference is whether or not the replacement teeth supported by implants are self-removable. Brånemark's first revolutionary implants were designed to be a permanent adjunct to the jaw and mouth, only removable by a dentist. Since then different types allow the patient to remove, clean and reattach their teeth to their implants on a daily basis. This is done by means of a snap fit or a clip bar. There are also hybrid configurations of these prostheses. We will describe each of these three choices in more detail in the third part of this book.

•39•

ARE IMPLANTS FOR YOU?

Physically speaking, not everyone is a candidate for dental implants. Psychologically too, a patience and discipline not always associated with our "quick fix" society are a much needed component in a successful implant regime. And finally, the financial factor is a reality which must be acknowledged. But stop and think about the car you're paying off. Implants too, provide comfort, pleasure, make you feel better about yourself, and allow you to live a less anxiety-ridden life. And properly done, this is one investment you will never have to replace or trade in.

Top: single right lateral incisor about to be placed on abutment which is attached to implanted fixture. Middle: Posterior teeth about to be placed over abutments which are attached to implant fixtures in the lower jaw. Bottom: Lower denture about to be placed over abutments which are attached to implant fixtures in lower jaw.

On the other hand, there are many physical and/or psychological conditions which frustrate osseointegration, most notoriously, tobacco's nicotine, which is unfriendly to the implant process. Still other dependencies including alcohol, heroin, cocaine, and pre-existing conditions like diabetes, cancer and its accompanying radiation therapy, autoimmune disorders or problems with circulation (usually accompanying diabetes) all lessen the chances of success to some degree. Further, pregnant women are discouraged from implant procedures, especially during the first three months. Additionally, it should be noted that certain mouth shapes require some surgical remodeling in order to accommodate implant placement, and the surgeon must make this decision.

•40•

Also consider that the personal cleaning of implants, like brushing natural teeth, is a daily requirement. It's for this reason that those with severe arthritis or other movement-inhibiting problems may prefer a different dental strategy.

We hope you're coming to appreciate that implants are a real commitment of time, money, and patience. Still, those with a "can-do" attitude can radically improve the quality of their lives through this procedure.

What Are the Unpleasantries?

Having said that, here is a list of the temporary unpleasantries known to accompany implant procedures in the first week following surgical procedures: temporary swelling and soreness of gums, discomfort from temporary bridge in the first weeks following first surgery; the limitations of a soft diet necessary in the first few weeks; and finally—withdrawal from tobacco, alcohol, and steak dinners.

Statistics show that patients who don't smoke or quit smoking for a crucial two week period (and best remain off tobacco for another seven weeks) have a far better success rate than smokers. Similar statistics exist for alcohol abusers, the reason being that nicotine and alcohol strip the mouth of enzymes vital to healing. We dentists hope the implant process can be looked upon as an enforced window of health, and will inspire a "clean regime" lasting long beyond the requirements of our specialty.

• 4 | •

Lastly, the long-term injuries which are a minute but undeniable possibility in implant procedures include: loss of bone mass if implants fail; bacterial infection stemming from the mouth or jaw; and minor nerve injury resulting in insensitivity or numbness to corner of mouth (a hazard of lower jaw implants only).

The Implant Fallacy:
Bad Press & Professional Jealousy

Because it took about 35 years for implantology to "grow up and become responsible," some stubborn doubts concerning its effectiveness persist. Also, among some traditional crown and bridge dentists, a reluctance to acknowledge a new procedure sometimes exists.

Obviously, patients with healthy teeth don't need implants, and do need the maintenance skills of conventional dentistry. But sometimes conventional treatment is less beneficial to long term success of the patient and so conventional dentistry should stand aside when a better alternative treatment is available. And to delay, detour, or prevent a client from seeking implant restoration as a solution to problems which clearly would be solved with such treatment would be most unfortunate, as well as immoral.

As we stated earlier, given a choice, natural teeth are always better than artificial ones. Unfortunately, it must be said that conventional dentistry is committed to certain practices which, when compared to implantology's alternatives, seem unfortunate. Specifically:

(1) To create a crown, a large portion of a live tooth is irretrievably ground away.

(2) To fit a denture plate on bare gums, all teeth—including some that may have years of potential use—are removed.

(3) Old-school crown and bridge techniques compromise the integrity of healthy teeth. This is perhaps the most unfortunate side effect of traditional treatment, since, when a tooth or group of teeth are damaged, conventional bridge techniques redistribute the pressure on neighboring teeth. It's like someone falling off a mountain being caught by another person they're tied to. The problem being: if the next person isn't perfectly positioned and very strong themselves, the first victim will drag a second victim with them. The same is true

of teeth. Nor is it long before you're involving a third for additional support, and then a fourth.

On the other hand, a single-tooth implant installed in the mouth early on in this scenario bolsters the health of its companion "natural" teeth. Since the implant relies solely on the jawbone for support, it makes absolutely no demands on other teeth (which are fatigued enough by stresses and strains of their own). Here is a clear case in which implantology totally assists conventional dentistry by protecting healthy teeth from undue strain. For while implantology is, by definition, an intrusive procedure, what we gain with a strategically placed single tooth implant can preserve existing teeth for years, even decades.

•43•

One Stop Shopping—Better Than A Specialist-by-Specialist Approach?

Perhaps you're beginning to recognize the fact that dental implants not only represent a huge step for you as a consumer, but also a daunting new step for dentistry the world over. Some dentists avoid the step, some master it, and some stumble attempting it. In certain dental offices often in the suburbs of large American cities, implants are spoken of casually, "Piece of cake. Sure we can. I took the seminar last weekend. Easy!" Don't ever place yourself in the care of people who tell you placing implants is easy.

In olden days, automobile companies such as Deusenberg and Bugatti would allow their customers to supply their own "coach-maker." The custom body would be mounted onto a chasis and engine by artisans of a completely different company, resulting in a completely unique automobile.

Similarly, some superior oral surgeons and periodontitis work in separate offices. These specialists begin the implant process, placing the original fixtures in bone, with no further involvement with their patients. Naturally, the marketplace abounds with restorative dentists who specialize in picking up the procedure from there. As specialists, their livelihood rests upon their reputations, and in a highly competitive field, many fine specialists obviously complete fine work in this manner. We prefer the advantages of a cooperative office because a second opinion, or a third or a fourth, is available in a matter of minutes. Without phone, fax, e-mail, secretaries, perhaps (if it can be believed!); without the use of anything but shoes on feet.

•44•

Also, there are some experts who "go it alone," though some might have a hard time believing that a single professional is equally adept in all three specialities of implantology, namely surgical, restorative, and laboratory. Sometimes their work is perfectly competent—sometimes not. But we ask you, what individual (aside from a modern day-Ben Franklin) could possibly compete with a team of specialists? The truth is that a cooperative office cannot help but result in superior troubleshooting, which means less bother, expense, and risk for you.

We're going to guess that "trouble-shooting" is not a word you're terribly comfortable with coming from dentists. Correct?

Because if we're so smart, then there shouldn't be any "trouble" to "shoot." Right? If all our scanners and X-rays-in-the-round don't tell us precisely how to do what we claim we're so good at doing, then why should there be any "trouble" doing it? This is a good question. With many answers. One of them being...

Implants are indeed bio-mechanical plants, and not every plant prospers. Take, for example, a patient who came to us 11 years ago with no lower teeth but with five implants placed in his jaw, one of which had failed to take proper root (or osseointegrate). We all met with the patient in a diagnostic session. It was clear that he needed a full bottom plate of 12 teeth. So we adjusted what would have been our strategy if all five implants had been healthy. Instead of installing a palateless denture (which requires five anchors), we installed the same number of teeth but fixed them into a traditional denture plate with a palate (which clips to a bar supported by four anchored abutments). After 11 years of use, this client is completely satisfied, even though his treatment began with a plan that changed due to an acknowledged single implant failure.

•45•

The best example of "trouble-shooting" is probably the consultation between professionals in placing and restoring implants—to illustrate this properly requires a brief technical explanation.

First Comes the Plan

Best results occur when implants are prosthesis driven. By this we mean that the task is to conceptualize a final fixture for your mouth which will solve all your dental problems, and then work backward from that design. With a final product in mind, we'll decide how many implants we need and where we need them. We'll hem and haw, discuss different ideas. The surgeon may suggest we should place one more implant than is absolutely necessary, as an insurance policy against possible loss. The dentist might warn of a particularly bad patch of gum infection at exactly the logical spot for the extra implant. The lab technician may suggest a different configuration of implants which solve both problems.

To be perfectly truthful, most every mouth we deal with is a whole little world of trouble. We earn your trust by doing the very best we can in that world. Indeed, it is our sworn duty, as well as the means by which we earn a living, to be the best we can be when we rehabilitate your mouth. You won't necessarily know it, but you—the patient—are our pride and joy. You are a walking monument to us. Sorry to be crass, but it's true. So it's vanity too, that drives a cooperative office—team spirit, even a hint of competition. Sure it's our livelihood, vocation, duty. Until finally, it is also our sincere pleasure to know that on a fairly regular basis, our work lessens suffering and creates greater opportunity for joy and comfort. So in a sense, yes, dentistry can actually be taken to a spiritual destination.

Indeed, we are here to serve you, even if "Trouble is Our Business." Because, as we began by saying: nobody walks into a dentist's office for fun. But while you're here you are our honored guest. And it is our great hope that when you leave, you'll leave as a friend.

CHAPTER TWO

A Visit-by-Visit Look at

IMPLANT

Procedures

Note: No two specialists are going to perform exactly alike, every mouth is different, and the number of implants needed will result in greater or lesser time—these are some of the reasons the "visit-by-visit" breakdown may vary from your implant experience. Also, in a cooperative office, consultations, observations, and even some procedural work by our surgeon and restorative dentist can be combined into the same visit.

Your First Visit: ARE YOU A CANDIDATE FOR IMPLANTS?

In Short:

Initial exam with restorative dentist and/or surgeon:

- medical history
- X-rays
- clinical exam
- diagnostic casts: models created from impressions of teeth (such casts will be made several times during the implant process)

TIME IN CHAIR: half an hour

RECUPERATION: none

In Depth: Dealing With Basic Hopes & Fears

Today—even with all the great things we can do—most people first walk into our office with apprehension most on their minds. What do they fear?

(1) pain

(2) injury

(3) expense

(4) losing huge chunks of time consumed by dozens and
dozens of dental visits.

What are their hopes? Why, what else but a set of teeth that
will make them look and feel like they once did, not so long
ago, when eating popcorn in the movies, laughing out loud,
and kissing your sweetheart was the right of every guy and gal.

So on the first visit, after we've had you fill out a health form,
taken new X-rays, examined your mouth thoroughly and made
diagnostic casts of your mouth, a restorative dentist will make
a dental evaluation, which means one of three things. You pass,
you don't pass, or you pass conditionally. (Meaning you have to
change something about yourself to qualify.)

•51•

If you pass, meaning that we've decided you and your mouth can
handle dental implants, you will most likely immediately return
to your initial fears. It's not your fault—it's human nature.

So quickly, let's address these issues:

As for Pain

We've explained that jawbones have much, much fewer pain
sensors than teeth do, which is why, depending on your health
and heartiness, we prefer to use a specific anesthesia in accom-
paniment with a mild sedative while performing first stage
surgery here in the office.

After first stage surgery the restorative dentist will fit you with a temporary bridge (or augment your old dentures) and recommend a diet of soft food which is mandatory for two weeks. Although you may not feel pain for the entire period, you must pamper the implants so that proper osseointegration can take place. From here on, for any psychologically stable person, the remaining procedures are considered pain-free.

Post-operative pain from the first stage fixture placement falls within tolerable limits, completely treatable with pain medications. The second stage surgery is even less intrusive and requires even less by way of anesthesia. Seven to ten days after the surgeon has placed healing caps on the bone integrated fixture, the restorative dentist is free to make the teeth which will be supported by the implant fixture.

What if Things Go Wrong?

We'd like to say that the days of implant failures are over, and compared to implantologies' rocky start—they are! But let the statistics speak for themselves. Implants succeed from 96% to 98% in the lower jaw, and from 89% to 94% in the upper jaw. It should be noted that this is statistically superior to almost any other medical procedure. For instance, hernia operations are between 30% and 40% unsuccessful, and must be redone if they fail. Understand too, that most of our cases meet with full satisfaction despite the rare instance of a single implant failure. Lastly, failed implants can be successfully replaced.

The most common problem associated with surgery is local infection. Secondly, any poorly executed bone-entering procedure can potentially damage nerves in the lower jaw. The worst case scenario, in the case of our specialty, would be loss of sensation in part of the mouth or a corner of the lip. Failed implants can also cause bone loss. Properly removed and cared for, the implant defect will re-fill with bone and gum, and become harmless in due time. Improperly removed or improperly treated, these bone defects can become infected. We also see a few cases of overgrowth of gums, although this is a far less serious and easily remedied complaint.

Finally, it should be noted that people with totally unrealistic expectations and/or severe psychological problems are risking the possibility of exacerbating these under the added stress of implant procedures, and such individuals might be best advised to seek other solutions to their dental needs.

•53•

THE COST

You will probably have to make a second visit to ascertain an accurate estimate of the full expense of a complete implant procedure. It wasn't so long ago that many very unhappy men and women would file into our office with naked hardware bristling from their gums. These were the victims of fast-talking "specialists" who convey the impression that they are providing full implant service, while in fact, they're merely placing a sped-up version of first and second surgery fast-tracked into one. It's a terrible thing to witness the faces of these people, most of them

old, many of them from foreign countries with a limited understanding of English. It's heartbreaking to see them cheated,
alienated, and confused. And it falls on us to tell them what a
full implant procedure will really cost. Assuming, that is, that
the work sprouting from their mouths is of serviceable quality.

The bottom line is that anyone considering a specialist-by-specialist treatment had better assemble a combination of at least
two separate bills, those of the surgeon and restorative dentist,
whose services include the lab work, before an approximation
of full costs can be accurately estimated.

About Insurance

Most patients automatically assume that implants are not covered by their dental insurance. What these individuals don't
realize is that a major component in the implant procedure,
is—of course—surgical, and is usually covered by dental and
medical insurance to some degree. A majority of dental and surgical offices feature an insurance expert on staff, who can pre-
certify your policy. If you have insurance, therefore, let the in-
office specialist make contact with your insurance company.
Just how a dental office contacts an insurance company has a
profound effect on what sort of response a given case will
receive; individual citizens are not always their own best advocates in these matters. Your specialist will portray your needs in
their best light, while keeping you fully informed of policy cov-
erage. This way, once a full cost estimate has been prepared,
you'll have a clear understanding of how much you, personally,

will be responsible to pay, over how long a period of time. Most people find the implant process a stressful period in their lives. If at all possible, do not compound this stress with the added anxiety of wondering, "However will I pay the bill?"

Costs and Payment Plans

Implant dentistry, like car purchases, is expensive. Both can be financed (and by the way…the dentistry lasts longer than the car). We dentists usually offer a care-credit plan which allows incremental payment for a year, and in some cases, two years—interest free.

A word on initial payment: some offices do and some offices don't charge for what we'll call, "the dental implant candidate exam," which is what this first visit basically amounts to. It's a tricky issue, and like most other things in this world, you get what you pay for. An office that doesn't charge for an exam may do a completely competent, honorable job. Then again, it is possible to lure in people of limited means with a "free consultation exam," and then "low-ball" the patient. By this we mean provide incomplete or misleading figures which represent only a portion of the final bill. Whereas an office that charges for an exam generally delivers a complete and comprehensive treatment plan. The irony being that this "expensive" dentist usually provides an estimate that falls on or below the final cost, while the guy who promises you a deal is more likely to pad the bill or use less costly implant components and a cheaper laboratory.

•55•

As for Time

Different types of implant restorations require different numbers of procedures, taking different lengths of time, and requiring differing periods of recuperation. This is why, for every type of procedure we describe, we'll also provide a recuperation table, as well as an estimate of how long you will be "in the chair."

Be an Educated Consumer

If you are a borderline candidate for implants, you might have to wait for test results before a verdict is reached. Nine out of ten individuals, however, will be told at their first appointment just where they stand. At the end of this first appointment, the would-be patient should be plainly informed of the gist of what we've just discussed and he or she should be given a rough cost estimate which will be fine-tuned on a second appointment.

A proper consultation will not:

- misinform or underestimate actual costs
- fail to inform you of the risks inherent to your case
- fail to address the realities of recuperation
- fail to inform you of how your treatment (and its cost) could be effected thereby.

CHAPTER THREE

A First

CASE

study

The first case we'll look at is for a patient with a single tooth that requires replacement. If the procedure is free of complications, the finished implant will be complete in eight to ten visits averaging less than an hour per visit. This will occur over a period as short as four months, with a first surgery recuperation period of about three months. Having said that, we should also note that a few short, painless check-ups which do not fall under a classifiable description are not at all uncommon in the business of trust.

Your First Visit: Meeting the Surgeon (or "Team")

In Short:

- diagnosis, treatment and financial plan
- should include information about risks and alternate strategies

TIME (NOT "IN CHAIR"): half an hour

In Depth: Consultation With Restorative Dentist & Surgeon

At the second appointment the surgeon will have a strategy in mind for you. An implant team will have already discussed your case in some detail, having come to some strong, though not final, decisions. The real business of the second visit is to fine-tune the plan. This is best accomplished when you meet the men and women who will be working together on restoring your mouth and discuss with them your questions and concerns.

If you are working specialist-by-specialist you should be as thorough in interviewing the restorative dentist as you are in interviewing the surgeon. In our office you get the benefit of these professionals advising each other; if you choose to deal with individual professionals, ask, ask, ask.

It is most important that you feel that your concerns are fully heard, thoroughly considered, and soundly answered. Doctor to patient, yes, but also human being to human being. If you get shy, however, and don't present real questions, it will be difficult to (a) really feel comfortable about the long, complicated procedure ahead, and (b) you may be inadvertently denying your hired "dental detectives" a full file with which to make extremely important decisions.

•61•

Look at the bulleted list which ends our description of the first visit, and make sure all parties involved—surgery, restorative, and lab—have fulfilled all these specifications. Do not worry about being polite, ask about pain, injury, money, time. And ask about alternative strategies (and the resulting change in cost) if you should encounter an implant failure. Important: get personal, talk about your eating and drinking habits, your public life, your private life, and any needs which may be specific to you. (One patient of ours, a college professor, decided he needed a removable bridge-plate because he had trouble lecturing in class if he had food in or under his teeth. With a bridge which clipped onto dental implants, however, he could "remove, rinse, and replace," after meals or even between classes—and his problem was solved).

Your surgeon, restorative dentist, and lab consultant should all view your panorex X-rays with you, collectively or individually. They will also show you an illustration of the type of implant configuration which has been tentatively chosen for you, and explain how the machinery will fit in your mouth, using models, drawings and X-rays. A second option may also be shown and discussed.

You may or may not be a candidate for a bone graft. If you are, make sure you've studied the chapter we dedicate to this quiet revolution. Be certain you're fully informed on any changes this could make on your recuperation, schedule and, of course, the bill.

You may have tooth impressions taken on a second visit. This time, however, the diagnostic cast will record the contours of the teeth across from the area to receive implants. In this way the lab can make an accurate model of "your bite,"—just how your upper and lower teeth meet—information which is crucial to a successful outcome. In the near future, the lab will create a perfect model of your mouth. Soon, hours of diagnostic work will be performed based on the model, without inconveniencing you—"the original."

Then a comprehensive treatment plan is presented, and that's about it for a second appointment. Again, you needn't necessarily want to marry your family off to these professionals, but you should get a sense that they are good at what they do, and take a measure of pride in providing real service. At the end of this visit your financial plan should have taken shape, which may or may not require a down payment. Make certain you understand the treatment plan and the proposed financial plan. For you will be responsible for following through with both these proposals.

TIME IN CHAIR: one half-hour
RECUPERATION: immediate

Your Second Visit: Stage I Surgery

In Short (At surgical office)

- implants surgically placed
- cover screws placed on implant fixture
- gums are closed
- diet, hygiene and medication reviewed

•63•

TIME IN CHAIR: depends on number of implants and whether any grafting takes place, i.e. a case-by-case situation.
RECUPERATION: 7-14 days for gums to heal, 4-6 months for implants to integrate

In Depth: Implant Placement

Assuming that extensive pre-implant bone grafts are not necessary, the very first surgical procedure opens locally anesthetized gums and reveals the significant section of jawbone. The procedure should be completed in a clean, closed environment, without rush or interruption. Some patients will have intravenous sedation, discussed with the surgeon at consultation. Ninety-five percent of patients will be conscious but sedated. The following is a description of surgery which some readers will, and some won't, wish to thoroughly familiarize themselves with. [For the technically minded.]

Revealing the Jawbone...

The surgeon will pre-drill the mandible (lower jawbone) at target spots along the crest of the gum's ridge with a guide drill. Then, with a slightly larger twist drill, he will insert direction indicators (which are like miniature surveyor posts) insuring proper depth, distance, and angle—parallelism of implants being crucial. He then repeats the process with larger (3.0mm) guide drill, twist drill, and direction indicators. (Gradually increasing the width of the canal insures precision and is less traumatizing to the bone.) He then countersinks a shallow area of greater width for second-stage hardware and first-stage screw cap.

Adding the Titanium Fixture

The site now properly prepared, the sterile, fully sealed titanium fixture is removed from its packaging and (with low-speed, perfectly calibrated, and vibration-free machinery) screwed into the bone. Hand-tools will finish the job, all of which have been precisely tested for proper torque. This fixture, threaded inside and out, is the titanium sleeve into which the abutment will be bolted in the second-stage surgery. Its hexagonal head is then covered with a temporary screw-down cap to prevent down

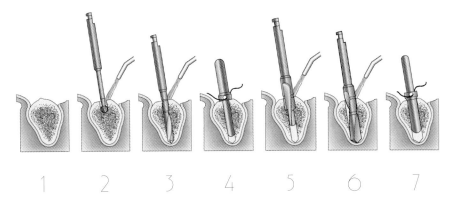

1) Undrilled jawbone. 2) First drill. 3) Twist drill into bone. 4) Post to a certain location. 5) Larger drill. 6) Larger still. 7) Final post measurement.

growth of soft tissue into the fixture canal. The cap is circular in shape and rounded on the top to be as "friendly" as possible to surrounding healing tissue. The cap also features a hollowed bullseye in the middle of its screw slot which will match the exploratory probe used at the beginning of second stage surgery. The bulls-eye is at the center of a hexagonal depression which will accommodate a screwdriver.

•65•

Time for Osseointegration

After the implant anchor (fixture) is set in bone the gums are stitched with removable sutures. The day after, your sutured gums will be swollen and sore. Use of prescription analgesics and antibiotics are routine for normal post-operative swelling and soreness, and to reduce a chance of infection. No denture of any kind is to be worn for 2 to 3 days. A soft diet is appropriate for a week or so. You must recognize that you'll endanger the entire procedure by placing any pressure on the post, and that no alcohol or tobacco is permissible, either.

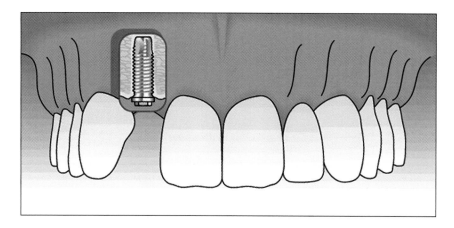

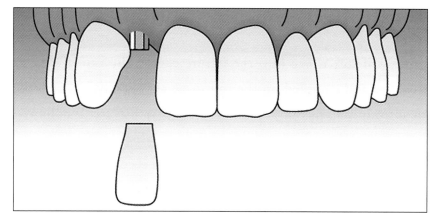

Implant fixture in the upper jaw at the site of the left lateral incisor.

TIME IN CHAIR: 1-4 hours (depending on number of implants)

OSSEOINTEGRATION PERIOD: 4 to 6 months.

YOUR THIRD VISIT: (at surgical or restorative office)

In Short: Follow-up to Stage One

- sutures removed
- surgical site evaluated
- denture or bridge inserted (depending on procedure)
- maintenance regime established

TIME IN CHAIR: 10 to 15 minutes
RECUPERATION: 4 to 6 months

In Depth: Post Operative

Ten to fourteen days after stage one, the surgeon will remove the sutures from your gums. The state of your healing process will be noted, and any post-operative complications (infection, tardy healing, etc.) are keenly watched for. A temporary denture (or your old denture newly adapted) will be lined with a soft material, and placed over your gums. Gentle, judicious chewing is henceforth permissible. It is customary for brief check-ups to follow every 6 to 8 weeks, two of which shouldn't take more than a half-hour.

TIME IN CHAIR: 10 minutes
RECUPERATION: on going, 4 to 6 months

Your Fourth & Fifth Visits
(At the restorative dentist office)

In Short:

Fast follow-up appointments to insure proper healing (Subsequent adjustment visits for temporary restorations may be necessary.)

TIME IN CHAIR: 15-30 minutes each
RECUPERATION: immediate

Your Sixth Visit:
Stage Two Surgery

(approx. 4 months after Visit #4 for lower jaw; 6 months after upper)

In Short:

- surgeon uncovers implants
- evaluation of osseointegration
- replace cover screw with healing caps
- adapting temporary denture/bridge to fit over healing cap
- surgeon now turns patient over to restorative dentist

TIME IN CHAIR: up to 1 hour
RECUPERATION: 3 to 7 days

•68•

In Depth:

First stage hardware is X-rayed to verify that proper osseointegration has taken place. After the gums are locally anesthetized, the surgeon's pin-probe identifies the exact center of the screw cap, and an incision is made revealing the fixture top. The rounded cap is removed. Cleaned and newly sterilized, the fixture now receives a healing cap, which protrude above the gum line and will train healing tissue to form around the abutment soon to follow.

The gumline is the horizon in implantology. The anchor is buried up to the gumline, and the abutment (which will support the prosthetic tooth) rises above the gumline.

The surgeon now sews the gum around the healing cap. In a successful implant process, this is the end of intrusive procedures. No further anesthesia or surgery will be necessary, and the restorative dentist will take over from this point forward.

TIME IN CHAIR: up to 1 hour
RECUPERATION: sutures to heal in 10 days

YOUR SEVENTH VISIT: MAKING A FINAL IMPRESSION

In Short: Post Stage Two Surgery

- impression coping placed onto implant
- mold is made of your mouth's new configuration (in preparation for the creation of final stage: finished teeth)

•69•

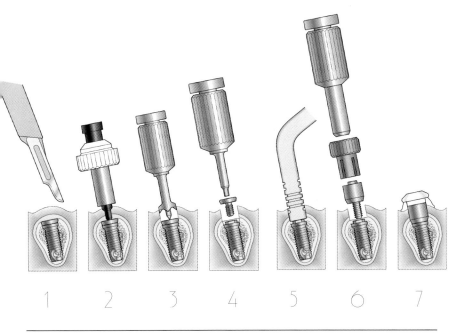

1) Uncovering the fixture in the bone. 2) Locating the healing cap. 3) Fine trimming the tissue around the healing cap. 4) Removing the healing cap. 5) Check of implant stability. 6) Placing the abutment. 7) Abutment in place with cap to protect it.

TIME IN CHAIR: 1 hour

RECUPERATION: immediate

In Depth:

After cleaning the healing cap, checking the overall hygiene of the mouth and finding you to be pain-free, the restorative dentist removes the healing cap and screws an impression coping or transfer assembly onto the implanted fixture "horizon" at gumline. A final impression is now made, upon which considerable lab work will depend. The impression coping is then replaced with the healing cap again.

TIME IN CHAIR: one and a half hours

RECUPERATION: on going

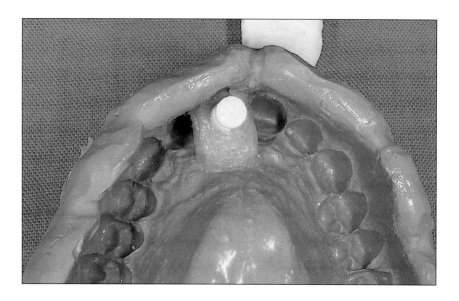

Soft tissue silicone material is applied to the impression around the abutment replica to simulate the contors of the gums when stone is poured into this master impression.

Meanwhile Back in the Lab...

In Short:

A model of the opposing jaw is set counter to the model of the implanted jaw. The lab and the restorative dentist designs its final restoration accordingly.

In Depth:

Once a full impression of the jaw with implant has been made, a "master model" is poured that perfectly replicates the patient's upper and lower jaws. An implant replica (called an "analog") is attached to the impression copings [see illustration]. Dental stone is now poured into the impression. Once the stone sets, the model is removed from the impression, creating an exact

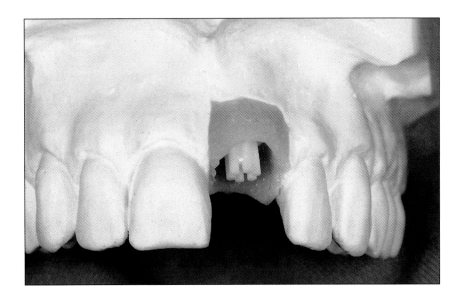

Master model with abutment replica and soft tissue.

duplicate of your dental arch with the analog in the exact position of the implant in your mouth.

Note: What follows is a description of basic mold techniques. The key to understanding molds is the realization that negative space in an impression becomes positive space in the mold.

The final impression of the mouth, including the part that we are restoring with a new tooth, is made with a pliable putty-like impression material. This remains true whether we are replacing a full arch of teeth, a quadrant or quarter of the upper or lower jaw, or a single tooth.

•72• The following is the procedure that takes place between your sixth and seventh visits. To recap visit #6: The healing cap which was placed approximately two weeks before by the surgeon, is unscrewed and removed, exposing the fully integrated implant fixture platform surface. At this time, a precisely machined transfer coping is placed into the implant fixture, locked over an external hexagonal part of the implant platform, and screwed into place.

Now, a precisely accurate putty impression is taken of the lower jaw. Once the impression sets firmly, it is removed from the mouth, sometimes (but not always) with the transfer assemblies (or copings) in place. These transfer assemblies are placed into the impression after being removed from the implant fixture in the jaw. At this time, the dentist or technician screws a replica of the implant fixture (the analog) onto the transfer assembly. The technician then pours a model of the implant fix-tures, duplicating the precise placement in the jaw. This is a first master model, which will have pink gums replicated, as well as any other "dental landmarks." It will be updated with all changes in your mouth.

Type of Implant

Aside from one exception which we will discuss later, all safe and up-to-date implant surgeries will follow these seven preliminary steps. Some offices will have more visits, some fewer, but the basic methodology is the same. We now find ourselves fast approaching the first "fork" in the implant road. Like the struc-ture of a "choose your own adventure," you will soon be invited to skip to the procedure appropriate to your specific case.

•73•

What Are Your Implant Needs?

Many of you know your problem, but some may not. Let us remind you that implants come in three basic configurations: single tooth, quarter jaw (three or four tooth), and full jaw. Unfortunately, dental difficulties do not always comply with such tidy remedies. Although this book cannot hope to replace a dentist, (do not attempt this at home!) we will, for educa-tional purposes, familiarize you with some of the more common solutions to problems we see over and over again.

1) Single lower left first molar being placed on abutment which is attached to fixture integrated into jaw bone. 2) Bridges being placed on abutments in lower jaw. 3) Hybrid denture that has been screwed into five abutments in the lower jaw.

NUMBER OF IMPLANTS...

A single tooth replacement, naturally, requires a single implant. Several single tooth replacements at different locations in the mouth, likewise, require as many single tooth replacements. If less than healthy teeth are outnumbered by severely compromised teeth, it may not make sense to preserve these few in an extensive rehabilitation. You may opt to have your entire dental arch replaced with implant supported teeth—a strategy which would entail "sacrificing" a few healthier teeth. However...

Note: Natural teeth keep circulation, gums, and bone mass healthier for the same reasons that a lived-in house, properly cared for, will age better than a shut-down, unheated neighboring structure. Similarly, for the overall health of your mouth it is preferable

•75•

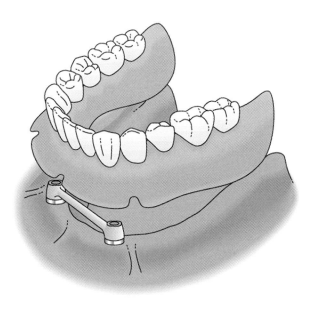

Two implants abutments joined with a bar onto which lower denture clips.

to keep as many natural teeth in your jaw as possible. One of the great advantages of implantology is that once osseointegration takes place, implant abutments can be adjusted to serve different purposes. Say, for instance, that four single tooth implants replace four doomed teeth in the lower jaw of a 60-year-old woman who gets nine more years out of her remaining natural teeth. At 69 she may have a full lower "clip on"(removable) bridge mounted on her four implants without any additional surgery, or she may have four additional fixtures implanted onto which a full set of permanent teeth will be fastened. (Remember, upper-class Americans are living to an average age of 86 among men, and 88 among women. Plan accordingly.)

•76• Two consecutive teeth in trouble should have two consecutive implants.

Generally three consecutive teeth also require two implants onto which we fasten a solid three-tooth bridge.

Likewise, four problem teeth will usually require three implant anchors. (A custom four-piece configuration could be made by a good lab technician, but this would be more expensive, and would require the same number of implants.)

Replacing five consecutive teeth usually requires four implant posts: two for a three-piece in the middle, augmented by two single tooth implants to either side or all joined.

KEEP IN MIND: With young or exceptionally sturdy bone structure, any configuration smaller than a half-mouth (quadrant) could be adequately supported with as few as three implants if these can be placed in a triangular configuration. When a comparatively small number of implants are going to withstand the forces placed on a comparatively large number of teeth, their anchors should be as far from each other as possible.

You should, by now, have a rough idea of what sort of implant strategy your lower jaw might require. The upper jaw is a trickier call due to differing anatomy and bone consistency. And while it's true that some of the logistics we've just used might be applicable, so many other variables must be factored in that it becomes unrealistic for a layman to "self-diagnose" with anything resembling accuracy.

•77•

BACK TO THE ACTION...

Fixtures successfully rooted, it's now time for the restorative dentist and lab technician to choose the middle stage in our three stage construction, namely the abutment. Let's continue our examination of the single tooth implant.

At this point we take the first of several impressions, beginning with a fixture-level impression of fixture, bone and surrounding gum. (At restorative visit #1.) Placing the preferred abutment onto the fixture in the mouth, we again cast a new, quite accurate mock-up of your mouth as it would appear with such an abutment in place. The lab and the restorative dentist now con-

fer, making certain that clinical as well as aesthetic requirements are fulfilled by this abutment arrangement in your jaw;
in some individual cases custom abutments may be fabricated.

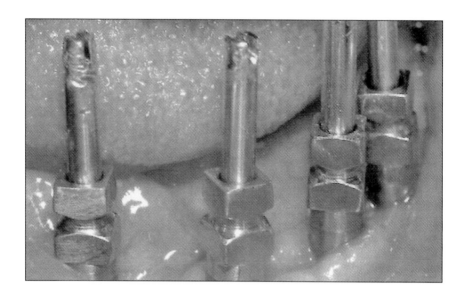

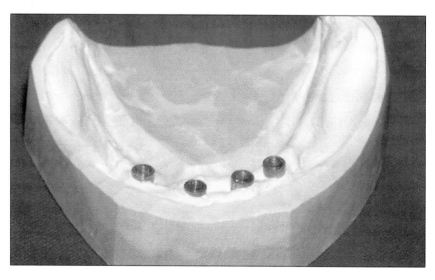

Top: Transfer assemblies attached to implant fixtures ready to be registered
with an impression. Bottom: Picture of master model of the jaw with fixture
replicas in place, ready to be used by lab technicians in fabricating dental
restorations.

Choosing the Hardware...

There are many different kinds of abutments for every possible case. Our office maintains a stock of hardware in excess of $40,000 in fixtures, abutments, and transfer assemblies for every foreseeable situation. Your dentist can order custom varieties of the above from the manufacturers if needed and will have the needed components the next day.

Having chosen the ideal abutment, the restorative dentist fastens it to the fixture to exact specifications. With one last abutment-level impression, the lab now makes a new master model. After establishing your bite and distance between jaws, a "perfect fit" is confirmed. This is accomplished by relating a separate stone model of your opposing jaw over the master model on a machine called an "articulator" which reproduces the chewing

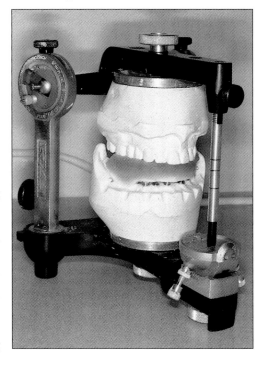

• 79 •

Mounted models on a semi-adjustable articulator replicating the upper jaw in relocation to master model with implant fixtures in place.

motion of your teeth at work. [See illustration page 79.] Thus, we have used the master model to replicate the placement of the implants, as well as the gums and jawbone around the implants. From this the lab can fabricate components, usually cast in a gold-palladium alloy. This casting is the frame upon which the final, most telling work begins—the part of the implant we see, use, and admire—the teeth. The lab usually starts this last phase with a cast made to fit the abutments or with abutment replicas fitted to our master casts.

Your Eighth Visit: Dress Rehearsal

In Short:

- a prototype is tried on for a fit
- a last check on "the new bite"
- selection of tooth "shade"

TIME IN CHAIR: 45 to 85 minutes
RECUPERATION: none

In Depth: The Framework Try-on

After fastening the prosthesis framework casting into your mouth, the restorative dentist will coat the top of the casting he has made with a bite registration paste. You'll gently, but firmly bite down, and this "jaw relation record" is removed. We then check this "new bite" against that established by the articulator and, if necessary, reposition the cast to match the upper teeth.

During this visit you will consult with the restorative dentist about shade and shape of your new teeth. Side mirrors and grid views of the face are sometimes used in selecting the size of the new set. The restorative dentist and the lab will by now have decided on very-near-the-exact position and angle of your new teeth.

This visit also provides the patient and doctor with the chance to make some last minute changes which will correspond with finalizing the perfect prosthesis. To take full advantage of this, several trial fits, with tiny adjustments after each, are not unusual or inappropriate. Coincidental to this last "try on," the paste-bite test will also be verifying jaw relation records, since the new tooth must mesh perfectly with "the old" or problems will eventually result.

Note: Since implants are connected directly to bone, they do not "give" like natural teeth do, resin-based prosthetic teeth absorb some chewing force, but not much. For this reason, we don't usually bridge a natural tooth to an implant. The natural one will move around, the implant won't, and the bridge may be compromised. Having said this, we also contravene this rule under specific circumstances too technical to discuss here.

Once you are completely happy with the aesthetics and "feel", the lab gets the green light to finish the final prosthesis, and the restorative dentist will replace your interim denture.

At the end of this "trying-on" session, the restorative dentist will replace the healing caps. These are still training new gum tissue to grow around what will soon be the finished hardware.

TIME IN CHAIR: 45 to 85 minutes
RECUPERATION: none

Meanwhile Back at the Lab...

Porcelain is baked onto the precious metal framework. This represents a "first bake," after which shade, shape, and bite will be adjusted.

•82• Your Ninth Visit: Restoration Completed

In Short:

- the final prosthesis will be screwed or cemented into place
- review of maintenance procedures [see special chapter]
- schedule for check-up appointments

TIME IN CHAIR: 45 minutes
RECUPERATION: none

INTERVIEW ONE

The subject is a 55-year-old female physician, who lives with her husband in Connecticut.

Q: Thank you for your patience in our game of phone tag, might I ask you about your dental history and what brought you to implants?

A: Well, I needed a single tooth replaced in my bottom teeth and as a matter of fact, once I heard you wanted to interview me I tried to remember which tooth it was and the strange thing is that it's been so seamless a procedure that I really don't know.

•83•

Q: You mean to say it's hard to know which teeth are real and which is the implant?

A: That's right.

Q: Amazing.

A: It is amazing. And it's a wonderful solution. Actually I'd considered having one in the upper jaw which is a more complicated operation involving moving the sinuses.

Q: It's called a sinus lift. It's a piece of cake, but back to your existing implant…Did you experience much pain and discomfort?

A: The happy thing is that there really was not much unpleas-
antness even at the time of surgery. I'd been anticipating
quite an ordeal, so I cleared the weekend and it wasn't necessary. I was fine the next day.

Q: Really? So the trauma was minimal?

A: That's right. I expected something like when I had my wis-
dom teeth removed, and it was nothing like that. They gave
me pain medication, and I didn't even have the black-and-
blue or much in the way of swelling which I'd been warned
about. I think mine was a particularly easy case.

Q: No black-and-blue jaw or swelling in the neck?

A: Neither. It was just an unusually successful procedure, I
guess.

Q: I guess so.

A: I mean, I'd heard terrible stories…

Q: Well, the old days of implants were something of a dark age.
But the new technology is amazing, and these particular
practitioners are pretty-damn good at what they do.

A: They're very good at what they do and they're also nice
people.

Q: I hear that again and again, but I'm not supposed to put it in the book. Tell me, was your problem just a case of normal attrition, no specific injury?

A: I don't have strong teeth, so it was—for me—normal wear and tear.

Q: Did the implant replace a bridge or a crown?

A: Yes, there had been a crown, but the root became too weak to support it properly.

Q: And how long ago was this done?

• 85 •

A: Maybe five years.

Q: And today you can't tell which is implant and which is real?

A: That's right.

Q: Well, it's not movie material—there's not enough drama in this story.

A: That's quite all right. I like it just the way it is. Thank you.

Q: Thank you.

CHAPTER FOUR

Front

TEETH

Your First Visit:
Are you a candidate for anterior implants?

In Short: Initial exam with restorative dentist and/or surgeon

- ascertain patient expectations
- medical history
- X-rays
- clinical exam
- diagnostic casts: models created from impressions of teeth (such casts will be made several times during the implant process)

TIME IN CHAIR: one half-hour

RECUPERATION: none

In Depth: General Overview of Anterior Implants

All healthy teeth grow from the gums at the crest of the ridge of both jawbones, likewise all implant fixtures are placed at this same ridge crest. In the rear, the ridge is wide, flat, and—particularly in the bottom jaw—deep, leaving the surgeon plenty of room to work. Also, rear teeth are not as visible, so from an aesthetic standpoint, the pressure to create porcelain works of art is somewhat diminished. All this changes in the "front row" of anterior restoration.

The frontal ridge crest of bone into which the surgeon must sink sturdy fixtures is steeper, narrower, and pointed. Appropriate implant sites are few. There is little or no room for error or experimentation. The surgeon must drill where there's sufficient

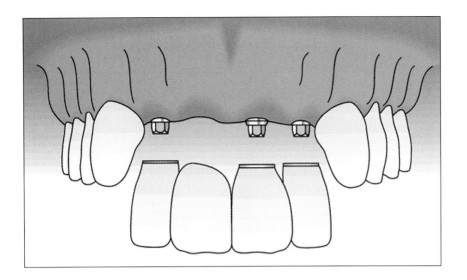

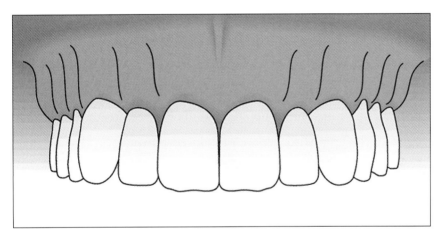

Top: Four-tooth bridge ready to be placed on three abutments which are attached to integrated implant fixtures. Bottom: Four-tooth implant supported with bridge in place.

bone, leaving it to the restorative dentist and the lab to finesse the rest. This job is made all the more challenging since front teeth, of course, are what a smile is all about. We are far more concerned about the appearance of our front teeth, nor is it only the teeth, proper, which concern us, but also the gum tissue which buffers the teeth (known as the papilla). The papilla rises and falls curtain-like, delicately delineating tooth from gum with a serrated edge much like the cuticle of a nail. There are some particularly tantalizing smiles (Whitney Houston and Goldie Hawn both come to mind) that capitalize on "exposed" papilla, wherein we witness the flash of teeth and what gives rise to the teeth all in one bold, yet-vulnerable, revelation.

So here—at the front of the mouth—we have the tightest constraints of surgery, coupled with the highest standards of personal aesthetics. In a removable clip-on restoration the papilla is fabricated, as is true of a traditional denture, but with permanent tooth or bridge implants the dentist must negotiate between the clinical needs of the surgeon and personal needs of the patient. Sometimes a sort of plastic surgery at the gum level is performed, this is where spot grafting can "plump up" the papilla between teeth. Or we may replicate the gum with a piece of colored porcelain.

These remarks hope to explain why the many "less crucial" visits will increase in number, the closer our procedures take us to the six front teeth. In this arena it is not unusual even for a romantic partner to be consulted before the final aesthetic decision is made. If you were considering body surgery or a hairpiece wouldn't it be the same?

It's important to realize that the teeth must be positioned where there is bone, thus occasionally, aesthetic compromises must be made. "The best that we can do,"(especially if we are working within cost constraints) may not be everything you want, cosmetically, but it will be all you need, dentally.

Your Second Visit: Meeting the Surgeon (or "Team")

In Short:

- diagnosis, treatment and financial plan
- should include information about risks and alternate strategies

TIME (NOT IN "CHAIR"): one half-hour
RECUPERATION: none

Your Third Visit: Stage One Surgery

In Short: (At surgical office)

- implants surgically placed
- cover screws placed on implant fixture
- gums are closed
- diet, hygiene and medication reviewed

TIME IN CHAIR: 1.5 hours
RECUPERATION: 7 to 14 days for gums to heal, 4–6 months for implants to integrate

Your Fourth Visit: (at surgical or restorative office)

In Short: Follow-up to Stage One

- sutures removed

- surgical site evaluated
- interim tooth, temporary denture or bridge inserted
- maintenance regime established

TIME IN CHAIR: 3/4 hour

RECUPERATION: (on going) 4 to 6 months

Your Fifth & Sixth Visits
(At the restorative dentist office)

In Short:

Fast follow-up appointments to insure proper healing

TIME IN CHAIR: 15–30 minutes each

RECUPERATION: none

Your Seventh Visit:
Stage Two Surgery

(approx 4 months after Visit #4 for lower jaw; 6 months after upper)

In Short:

- surgeon uncovers implants
- evaluation of osseointegration
- replacement of cover screw with abutments upon which healing caps are placed
- modification of temporary denture to fit over healing abutment/healing cap
- surgeon now turns patient over to restorative dentist

TIME IN CHAIR: up to one hour

RECUPERATION: sutures to heal in 10 days

YOUR EIGHTH VISIT:
MAKING A FINAL IMPRESSION

In Short: Post Stage Two Surgery

- impression coping placed onto implant
- mold is made of your mouth's new configuration (in preparation for the creation of final stage: finished teeth)

TIME IN CHAIR: 1 hour

RECUPERATION: immediate

•93•

MEANWHILE BACK AT THE LAB...

In Short:

A model of the opposing jaw is set in opposition to the model of the implant jaw. The lab designs its final restoration accordingly.

YOUR NINTH VISIT:
DRESS REHEARSAL

In Short:

- a cast framework is tried in for a fit
- a last check on "the new bite"
- selection of tooth "shade"

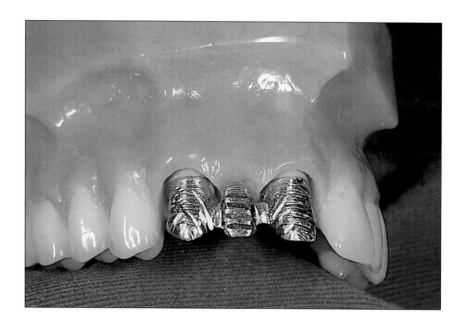

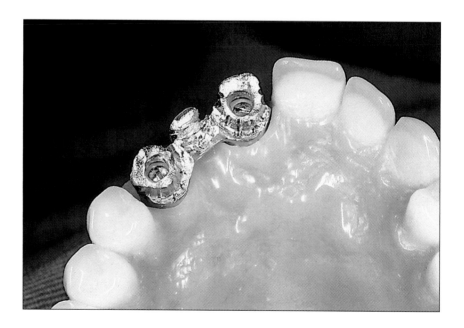

Top: Cast framework on model. Note the perfect fit of the margins to the shoulders of temporary cylinders. Bottom: Palatal view of cast framework on model.

TIME IN CHAIR: 45 to 85 minutes

RECUPERATION: none

MEANWHILE BACK AT THE LAB...

Porcelain is baked onto the precious metal framework. This represents a "first bake," after which shade and shape will be adjusted.

YOUR TENTH VISIT:
RESTORATION COMPLETED

IN SHORT:

- the final prosthesis is screwed or cemented into place
- review of maintenance procedures [see special chapter]
- schedule for check-up appointments

•95•

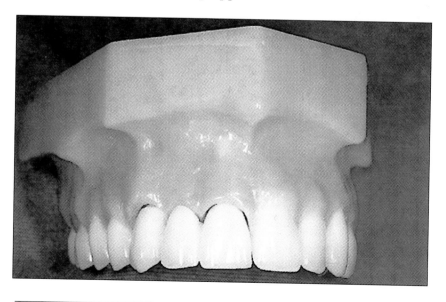

Above: Finished screw-retained cast-framework restoration ready for insertion.

TIME IN CHAIR: 45 minutes

RECUPERATION: none

INTERVIEW TWO

The subject is a 19-year-old woman enrolled in a New England liberal arts college. Her mother told us the worst thing about her daughter's implants was driving into the city at rush hour for the appointments. Then she gave us her daughter's phone number.

Q: Could you tell me what happened to you that caused you to have implants placed at such an early age?

A: I had teeth pulled by my orthodontist to make room for braces when I was 15. I guess they tried to move the teeth too fast, and what happened was they cut off the roots to two other teeth.

Q: That's awful.

A: Yeah.

Q: Which ones were they?

A: The top teeth to either side of my two front teeth. Incisors, they're called.

Q: Got it. Go on.

A: Well those two teeth were just like hanging there, so we had to have them pulled and have the dental implants done.

Q: Now with the surgeries, did you have any problem with them? Did you have much pain?

A: No, I really didn't have any problem with them. There was some pain, like, right after them but that was expected.

Q: And what about temporaries? Did you have a different set made for between the surgeries?

A: Yes, I had two sets made. I went to sleep-away camp and had two sets—just in case one broke.

•97•

Q: I see. So the whole experience lasted how long?

A: I was just 16 when I had the first surgery, and six months later I had the second surgery.

Q: So that must have been difficult at 16.

A: Yeah, having the temporaries made it the most difficult. You know, walking around with fake teeth in your mouth when you're a kid is a bit weird, not telling your friends and stuff, cause they'll tell other people…it's weird.

Q: And so now you've got permanent ones?

A: Yeah.

Q: So when you run your tongue over them they feel normal?

A: Yeah.

Q: Well, that's a good thing. You know your doctor told me he hasn't seen you for a yearly cleaning. Did you know you're supposed to go once a year?

A: Oh, I guess I forgot.

Q: I mean, he's glad you haven't had any problems but he did ask me to remind you.

A: OK, I'll tell my parents when I go home for Thanksgiving.

Q: So this is your freshman year?

A: Yeah, it's my first year—it's hard too.

Q: But at least you don't have to worry about your smile being weird.

A: That's true. I definitely don't need that problem on top of everything else. Hey, do I get a copy of this book?

Q: Sure.

In case you're suspecting we've only chosen "perfect cases," here is a quick interview with a physician in his late 50s who had some difficulties.

INTERVIEW THREE

Q: Could you give me a quick dental history and what brought you to resort to implants?

A: Well, I had two broken front lower teeth from an accident, which were capped for some time but the caps did not really work very well and kept falling off and breaking. Finally, Dr. Wiland decided that I would be a good subject for implant surgery. I had the surgery with his colleague who was an excellent surgeon. Not merely competent technically, but was also excellent with people; he explained what would be done and the surgery was handled very well. There were follow-ups which alleviated some discomfort, and I was also kept informed as to our progress.

•99•

Q: Now were there some peculiar circumstances or was this the traditional two-step surgery?

A: There was one unusual circumstance…let me tell it my own way.

Q: Go ahead.

A: I've been under the care of Dr. Wiland for many years. His technical expertise coupled with his sense of aesthetics are, together, really quite remarkable. He fashioned two false teeth which I used between the implant surgeries so I was able to function normally, and then when the work was done and the implant finished it was fitted and adjusted and worked very well. Unfortunately, at one point there was a screw that did break, which is not a function of dental skills, but the frailty of a piece of a mechanical hardware that can fail under the best of circumstances. Dr. Wiland was cognizant of all this and explained it all to me and sent me to a colleague who, with a kind of electric microscope, was able to remove the damaged screw, and shortly thereafter a new one was put in which served the purpose quite well and I've had no difficulties since then.

Q: So the temporary false teeth which you wore between the first and second surgeries—those then were adjusted to become the permanent prosthesis?

A: No. The temporary ones fit over the gums, they were there for aesthetics and so I could eat. I was able to carry on with my professional work which includes a lot of speaking. Then when the final prosthesis was ready the temporaries were discarded.

Q: I understand.

A: Then the adjustments took place and it was very gratifying.

I have no regrets, as a matter of fact, I'm very pleased with the way it looks and the way it feels and that I can carry on my normal life unaware that I have anything in my mouth other than my own teeth.

Q: So these are not removable.

A: These are permanently installed. They can be removed for cleaning once a year. Two teeth on two posts. And that's what I have to say. Does that help you?

Q: Yes it does. One last question: Did you have any pain during the healing process?

A: During the surgery itself there was no pain, but during the healing process there was some pain because evidently where the teeth had been removed and the implants inserted, there was a certain amount of gum healing, which was not so much painful as, shall we say, bothersome, for a short period of time. But I think that's part and parcel of any surgery, but once it healed I had no difficulties.

CHAPTER FIVE

Full Lower

ARCH

Replacement

In Short:

Initial exam with restorative dentist and/or surgeon

- medical history
- X-rays
- clinical exam
- diagnostic casts: models created from impressions of teeth (such casts will be made several times during the implant process)

TIME IN CHAIR: one half-hour

RECUPERATION: none

In Depth:

Let's look at a patient with no bottom teeth. The implant chosen for this case is called "a bar-retained mandibular over-denture supported by implants," which means, in plain language, a user-removable plate fit with a full set of bottom teeth which snaps on a bar of two or more posts where the bottom front teeth once were. If the procedure is free of complications, the finished implant-supported denture will be complete in ten visits, averaging less than an hour per visit. This will occur over a period as short as five months, with a first surgery recuperation period of about four months. Having said that, we should also note that a few short, painless check-ups which do not fall under a classifiable description are not at all uncommon.

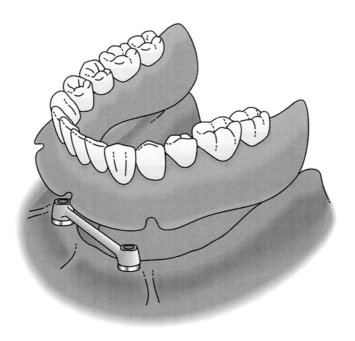

Lower denture being placed on abutments that are attached to bar onto which denture clips.

Your Second Visit: Meeting the Surgeon (or "team")

In Short:

- diagnosis, treatment and financial plan
- should include information about risks and alternate strategies

Time (not in "chair"): one half-hour

Recuperation: none

Your Third Visit:
Stage One Surgery

In Short: (At surgical office)

- implants surgically placed
- cover screws placed on implant fixture
- gums are closed
- diet, hygiene and medication reviewed

TIME IN CHAIR: 1.5 hours

RECUPERATION: 7 to 14 days for gums to heal, 4-6 months
for implants to integrate

Your Fourth Visit:
(at surgical or restorative office)

In Short: Follow-up to Stage One

- sutures removed
- surgical site evaluated
- interim tooth, temporary denture or bridge inserted
- maintenance regime established

TIME IN CHAIR: 3/4 hour

RECUPERATION: (on going) 3 to 5 months

Your Fifth & Sixth Visits
(at the restorative dentist office)

In Short:
Fast follow-up appointments to insure proper healing

TIME IN CHAIR: 15-30 minutes each
RECUPERATION: none

Your Seventh Visit:
Stage Two Surgery

(approx 4 months after Visit #4 for lower jaw; 6 months after upper)

In Short:

- surgeon uncovers implants
- evaluation of osseointegration
- replacement of cover screws with abutments upon which healing caps are placed
- modification of temporary denture to fit over healing abutment/healing cap
- surgeon now turns patient over to restorative dentist

•107•

TIME IN CHAIR: up to 1 hour
RECUPERATION: sutures to heal in 10 days

Your Eighth Visit:
Making a Final Impression

In Short: Post Stage Two Surgery

- impression coping placed onto implant fixture
- mold is made of mouth's new configuration (in preparation for the creation of final stage: finished teeth)

TIME IN CHAIR: 1 hour
RECUPERATION: immediate

Meanwhile Back at the Lab . . .

In Short:

A model of the opposing jaw is set counter to the model of the implant jaw. The lab and the dentist design their final restoration accordingly.

Your Ninth Visit:

In Short:

- abutment level impression is taken (a.k.a. "master model")
- opposing jaw model is made
- final framework is cast

TIME IN CHAIR: one half-hour
RECUPERATION: none

Your Tenth Visit:
Dress Rehearsal

In Short:

- cast framework is fitted
- a last check on "the new bite"
- selection of tooth "shade"

TIME IN CHAIR: 45 to 85 minutes.
RECUPERATION: none

Meanwhile Back at the Lab...

A denture is made to fit over framework.

Your Tenth & Final Visit:
The Final Prosthesis

In Short:

The bar framework is screwed onto the abutments in your mouth and the denture is clipped onto the bar.

- review of maintenance procedures [see special chapter]
- schedule for check-up appointments

TIME IN CHAIR: 45 minutes

RECUPERATION: none

In Depth:

Visit #10 will involve a gold or gold-palladium alloy bar being fastened on the titanium uprights. The finished denture plate will clip onto the bar, and aside from checking for comfort and "the bite," treatment is complete. It is now up to you to fulfill your responsibility of keeping a series of check-ups and learning how to clean the plate, clip and bar. Another type of self-removable plate involves pressure activated ball-and-socket clips, not unlike clothing "snaps."

Remember: Extensive maintenance is required of this type of implant support. Cleaning is crucial to success! [See chapter on Maintenance.]

1

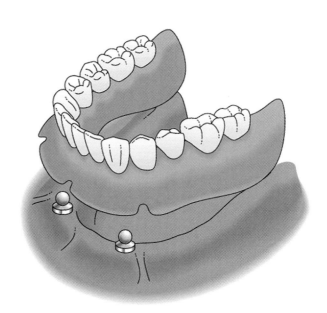

2

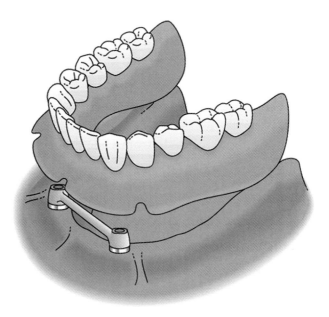

1) Full lower denture being placed on ball attachments supported by implants.
2) Full lower denture being placed on clipbar supported by implants.

3

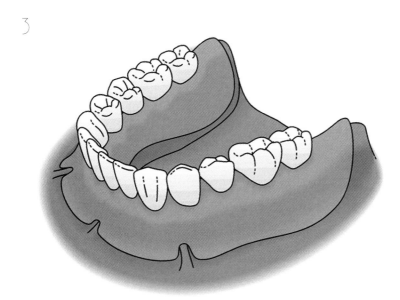

4

• | | •

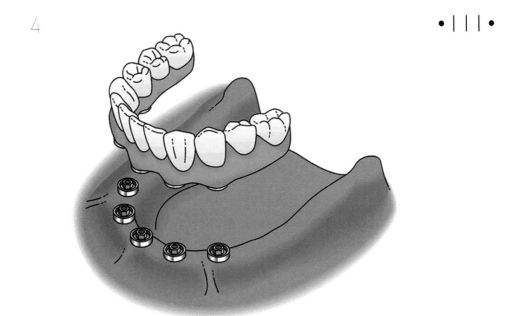

3) Full lower denture securely in place and able to be removed by patient.
4) Full lower denture being placed by screwing the denture onto five integrated fixtures with abutments and can be removed by dentist.

By now you now have sufficient understanding of the implant process to appreciate the three main families of present-day implants.

(1) The single tooth replacement implant is removable only by a dentist, and is fastened to the implant fixture at or slightly below the gumline. It is not a denture and most closely resembles a natural tooth.

(2) A hybrid denture, which comes in a full or partial arch, is screwed into abutment supports at or slightly above the gumline and is removable only by a dentist.

(3) A clipbar or ball-and-socket denture which also is created as a full arch or partial arch and is removable by patient.

All three of these configurations are installed in a three stage procedure, the first two of which are surgical. We:

(1) implant fixtures;

(2) fashion a support system;

(3) create a restorative prosthesis which is mounted on this support system (which in turn is mounted on the fixture).

The means by which we install the finished teeth comprise the three families of implants discussed in the previous chapter.

INTERVIEW FOUR

The subject who is an art historian from the U.K. in his early forties, has compromised bone quality and limited funds. Due to his financial situation, we did not perform bone grafting.

Q: Can you tell me what brought you to implants?

A: I've got bad teeth—always have. One dentist wanted to pull them out and put in false ones, but I couldn't go for that. Vanity, you know? So I heard about implants a while back but I couldn't afford them. Then I got a job with a partial dental plan. In my line, you've got to take what you can get.

Q: So you saw the opportunity to have implants put in and jumped for it.

A: That's right. As a Christmas present to myself in '97. I had three put in. Lost one. I blame it on lousy diet—too little calcium. But that's me Mum's fault and a whole other story.

• | | 3 •

Q: The upshot is: you had three implants put in and you lost one.

A: That's right.

Q: Was there much pain?

A: No, just a lot of waiting, which is pain enough.

Q: Were you a smoker?

A: Was and still am, sorry to say. I went on the patch for the surgery—which was a blessing.

Q: And alcohol?

A: Yeah, there was a crucial two week period there when I think I had two beers the whole time.

Q: So your dental strategy was adjusted to accommodate three implants reduced to two?

A: That's it. They did just fine with the two. I got a lower plate that snaps on and off with a ball-and-socket system—so I can clean the food out from under the plate between lunch and my next meeting.

Q: Was that system cheaper than the unremovable—or I should say "dentist removable" system?

A: Yeah, I believe it was a bit cheaper.

Q: You mind if I ask how much it was?

A: All in all, it was about $11,000, and I paid half. Now I'm saving up for the uppers.

Q: I guess that means you're happy with the results.

A: That's right. With the mess I walked in with…I'm very happy with new teeth—but I haven't put them to the true test.

Q: And what's that?

A: A barroom brawl. Just joking!

CHAPTER SIX

Full Upper

ARCH

Replacement

Your First Visit: Are You a Candidate for Implants?

In Short:

Initial exam with restorative dentist and or surgeon

- medical history
- X-rays
- clinical exam
- diagnostic casts: models created from impressions of teeth (such casts will be made several times during the implant process)

TIME IN CHAIR: one half-hour

RECUPERATION: none

In Depth: General Overview

Implants in the upper jaw, or maxilla, are more difficult to perform, take longer to heal, and have a slightly lower success rate than mandible, or lower jaw, implants. The maxillary bone which delineates the floor of the sinuses is spongier and of less consistent height. If it is ten millimeters or more, an implant process much like the one already described proceeds, often accompanied with simultaneous spot bone grafting, which much resembles the repointing of an old chimney.

If the maxilla is less than ten millimeters, a preparatory bone graft or "sinus-lift" becomes first priority. This entails tucking the sinus membrane higher into the sinus cavity making available to our surgeon stronger, healthier bone higher up the face. In older patients, with whom tooth loss and root breakdown is common, such comparatively fresh bone can be used for grafting elsewhere in the mouth—without a further "harvesting" wound in the leg or rib.

Compared to full lower arch replacement, full upper arch replacement is a more complex, more expensive and a potentially more stressful procedure. However, by familiarizing yourself with the following step-by-step procedure, you should be able to anticipate what is involved and be better prepared to deal with its ramifications.

Your Second Visit: Meeting the Surgeon (or "Team")

In Short:

- diagnosis, treatment and financial plan
- should include information about risks and alternate strategies

TIME (NOT IN "CHAIR"): one half-hour
RECUPERATION: none

In Depth: Sinus Lift

The main diagnostic decision for full upper arch replacement is whether or not to perform a sinus lift. Let's look briefly at a sinus lift procedure and then continue our breakdown. Such a procedure takes about an hour and a half to perform. It can accompany implant fixture placement (when sufficient bone is revealed by the lift); it can also accompany spot grafting in addition to fixture placement [see Bone Grafting chapter]. In extreme cases, in which many centimeters of bone must be prefabricated before implant placement, the lift becomes a separate procedure requiring a recuperation period of approximately six months. Between 10 and 13 millimeters of bone is preferred for fixture placement in this region. A sinus lift will not cause a sinus condition, nor exaggerate pre-existing sinus conditions—these are associated with the upper sinuses. We have never performed nor heard of a sinus lift "failure."

Your Third Visit: Stage One Surgery

In Short: (At Surgical Office)

- implants surgically placed
- cover screws placed on implant fixture
- gums are closed
- diet, hygiene and medication reviewed

TIME IN CHAIR: one and half hours
RECUPERATION: 7 to 14 days for gums to heal, 4-6 months for implants to integrate

Your Fourth Visit: (At Surgical or Restorative Office)

In Short: Follow-up to Stage One

- sutures removed
- surgical site evaluated
- interim tooth, temporary denture or bridge inserted
- maintenance regime established

TIME IN CHAIR: 3/4 hour

RECUPERATION: (ongoing) 4 to 6 months

Your Fifth & Sixth Visits
(At the restorative dentist office)

In Short:

Fast follow-up appointments to insure proper healing

TIME IN CHAIR: 15-30 minutes each

RECUPERATION: none

Your Seventh Visit:
Stage Two Surgery (approx 6 months after Visit 4)

In Short:

- surgeon uncovers implants
- evaluation of osseointegration
- replacement of cover screws with abutments upon which healing caps are placed
- modification of temporary denture to fit over healing abutment/healing cap
- surgeon now turns patient over to restorative dentist

TIME IN CHAIR: up to 1 hour

RECUPERATION: sutures to heal in 10 days

YOUR EIGHTH VISIT:
MAKING A FINAL IMPRESSION

In Short: Post Stage Two Surgery

- impression coping placed onto implant(s)
- mold is made of your new implant fixtures (in preparation for the creation of final stage: finished teeth)

TIME IN CHAIR: 1 hour

RECUPERATION: immediate

YOUR NINTH VISIT:

In Short: Creating the Master Model

- we take an abutment level impression (a.k.a. "master model")
- also take an impression of the opposing jaw

MEANWHILE BACK AT THE LAB...

In Short:

A model of the opposing jaw is set in opposition to the model of the implant jaw. The lab designs its final restoration accordingly.

Your Tenth Visit: Dress Rehearsal

In Short:

- a framework is tried in for a fit
- a last check on "the new bite"
- selection of tooth "shade"

TIME IN CHAIR: 45 to 85 minutes

RECUPERATION: none

•123•

Meanwhile Back at the Lab . . .

Porcelain is baked onto the precious metal framework. This is a "first bake," after which shade and shape will be adjusted.

Your Eleventh Visit: Restoration completed

In Short:

- the final prosthesis is screwed or cemented into place
- review of maintenance procedures [see special chapter]
- schedule for check-up appointments

TIME IN CHAIR: 45 minutes

RECUPERATION: none

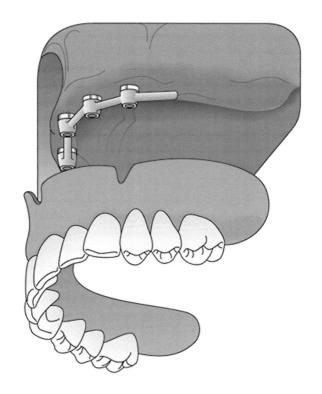

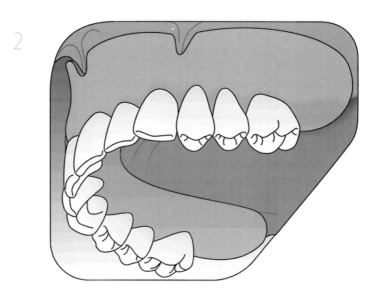

1) Upper palateless denture being clipped onto implants supported bar that is attached to implant abutments. 2) Upper palateless denture clipped into bar and in place.

3

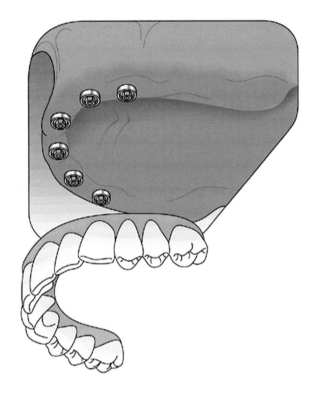

4

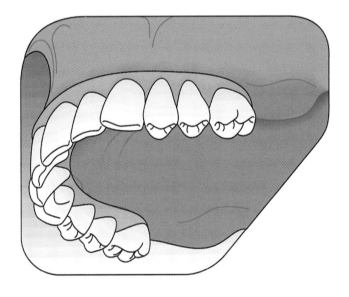

3) Upper palateless denture ready to be screwed into place. 4) Upper palateless denture screwed into place.

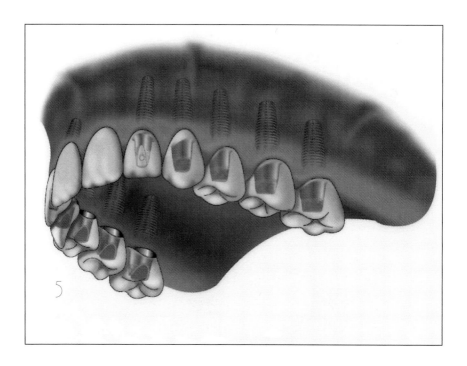

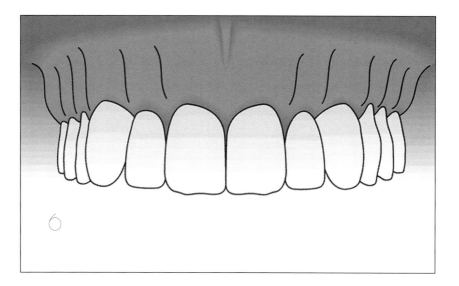

5) Front tooth bridge with four teeth ready to be screwed into three abutments which are attached to fully integrated implant fixtures. 6) Upper fixed bridge screwed into place.

Interview Five

The subject is a nurse who works in the greater New York area.

Q: What dental problems brought you to implants, and how did you decide to commit yourself to an implant program?

A: I lost three teeth, and I never knew I had gum disease. No one ever said the word "gingivitis." Then I went to have my teeth cleaned, and the hygienist said, "Oh yeah, you have a little bit of gum disease. Nothing to worry about…" And that office referred me to another office, the same old story, and it wasn't long before I lost another tooth.

•127•

Q: And no one was being straight with you about that. Like losing four teeth was business as usual?

A: That's right. They just said I had "bad teeth." So I'd get a root canal, then they'd put a cap on it. Then the root would die, and before you know it, they'd say "It's got to come out."

Q: And you feel there was some deceit in this?

A: Let's just say the patient is the last to know…and while I'm in the dark, I'm writing lots of big checks and going through a lot of pain and fear without ever really knowing the truth—I have gum disease. I didn't have "bad teeth." I had diseased gums. So I'm on the way to losing, I think, my fifth tooth and I'm freaking out, but my newest dentist is saying: "Don't worry, go to this specialist, he works miracles." So I go, he says I need braces. He says by moving my teeth over a little he can get them rooted to stronger bone. So, unfortunately, I listen to him. And then my problems really began.

Now I happen to meet a guy who works in dentistry who I have come to trust on a personal level, and I say to him: "I don't want to be your patient, but I need to know the truth about what's happening in my mouth." So he refers me to your office. I know you don't want an ad campaign, but the truth is I was desperate. So Dr. Wiland saw me, took X-rays, then he called a periodontist in for a consultation. And they told me: every tooth has to go. Couldn't believe it. EVERY TOOTH HAS TO GO. Of course, I said, "No way." And then the periodontist said, "If you insist on holding onto those teeth, I won't take you on as a patient." And that, awful as it was to hear, was the first time I got let in on the real deal. Rather than being told everything would be all right and to just keep signing checks, I was told: "Your mouth is a complete and total disaster."

Q: Do you mind if I ask how old you were when you were told this?

A: I was 40.

Q: So you're 40 years old and you're told you have to have every tooth in your mouth pulled? I would have cried. Did you?

A: As a matter of fact I did, a little. I got very quiet, and just kind of closed down, but then they said, "But the good news is we can fix this." Now you have to understand I'd been told, "Don't worry, we can fix this" quite a few times already, and I don't even know if I totally believed it. But the fact is I was desperate, and it's like anything else—no matter how many times you've been let down, you've got to find a reason to trust again.

Q: So this was the first time you heard about implants?

A: Well, I was upset, and they were very comforting and they said, "We've got to work out a game plan. There's a step by step procedure that will give you pain-free, worry-free tooth replacements. Not dentures. Although you'll wear them briefly." And I guess that's when I first heard the word implants, but I don't really remember. I was numb. And to tell you the truth I didn't realize the amount of time it would take, o.k.? Not until we actually started. I sort of went blank—like ignorance is bliss—lucky for me I didn't end up with another bunch of shysters, they could have put a nuclear bomb in my jaw and told me my last appointment was in the World Trade Center, and I'd have blown up New York. I mean it! Sorry—no, of course, they told me, about a two stage surgery, with a long healing stage in between. But I was in the twilight zone. I've seen it a hundred times because I work in the health-care field, a patient gets to a certain point and it just goes in one ear and out the other...Numbers, dates, prices. Forget it, they're in a deep

• 129 •

freeze. But like I said, I finally got lucky. It was unbeliev-able. They gave the bad news first, and from that point on it only got better. Right up through surgery. And the sur-geon calls me the next day, I couldn't believe that. Then they told me the waiting is worst. And it was.

Q: Between first and second surgeries, you mean.

A: Right. You get restless, you get disgusted—it's true. Everyone says, "You're not done yet?"

Q: Like your boyfriend in particular.

A: (*Laughs*) Yeah, right.

Q: So how bad was the surgery, were you aware of cutting and the like?

A: Actually—and this is strange—it was a breeze for me. I'm going to tell you something, when I went to the dentist I used to get sick and get so upset and I started taking Valium. But when I went into the appointment for surgery—I tell you the truth—I didn't get upset. I just got a little fidgety, you know? Like, I don't really want to sit there for an hour and a half. But the big-time panic is, like, gone.

Q: And you were semi-conscious during the operation?

A: Yeah, it's fabulous the way they do it. They put a little intravenous in your arm and in a matter of seconds you're
twilight…You kind of hear things in the background but
you're not really present. In the first one, the biggie, I got
up in the middle of it. You know, I guess I didn't quite know
what was going on. It seems they replaced a fair amount of
bone that holds in my teeth. I got a little frustrated with
something or other, and I just got up to leave. It's pretty
funny really. I had a girlfriend who had the same reaction
having a baby—like—enough of this action, I'm going
home. The doctors have to remind you what's going on.
Talk you back down. So when all was said and done, the surgeon asked me how long I thought the procedure took. I
said, "Fifteen minutes." He laughed and said, "Try three
and a half hours."

• | 3 | •

Q: Wow. This was top or bottom or both?

A: Just the uppers. I know enough about recuperation not to
overload my system, I'd rather have a longer recuperation,
go in a second time, even spend a little more money on the
extra procedure than to have both top and bottom done at
once. Your system gets fairly traumatized as it is.

Q: So you had a fair amount of bone grafting done, right?

A: That's right. At one point I heard him say that my teeth
were literally held in with soft tissue. There was no bone
left. So they replaced it. First they drew blood from one

arm, and then they isolate your platelets, and they mix it with this artificial bone. And they pour that in and replace my bone, and then they laid the abutments in that.

Q: You know your stuff.

A: You know what? It reminds me of construction. I've got in-laws in construction. You know—they mix up the concrete, then pour the foundation, then lay the ironwork in the concrete and then bingo—you put in your beam and you can screw and nail to that…build the house.

Q: Hey, you wanna write this stuff for me?

A: That's ok. I got my work cut out for me.

Q: No pun intended. Next question…Do you consider yourself a person with low, normal or high tolerance to pain?

A: I'm tolerant of pain, I'd have to say. But that's physically …psychologically, no. I've had oral surgery before where I was sick as a dog with much less surgery than this. And it was from worry. These guys give you instructions when you leave, and you follow these instructions. You're told exactly what's going to happen, so you don't panic. You go home afterwards. You take your pain pills before the anesthesia wears off and you sleep it off. Seventy-two hours later you swell, twenty-four hours later it goes down. Maybe I was a textbook case, but what happened to me was exactly what they'd written out. And what's more they called me the night of surgery, they're always available, and let's face it— that puts your mind at ease. I've had surgeries where you call up and the surgeon is in the Bahamas. Hello, goodbye.

Q: So that's surgery and post-op…Now did they fit you with temporary dentures?

A: Yes, they did. They left four teeth because I couldn't deal with a removable plate. You know, taking your teeth out to clean them? I wouldn't do it. I've got a thing about that. I worked in an E.R. for a long time as a nurse's aid, and whenever these people come in with respiratory arrest, cardiac arrest, the first thing you do is whip out the teeth. And I always ended up with the job of finding their teeth, and it's just permanently creeped me out around dentures. So they left the four best teeth to anchor a temporary bridge around.

•133•

Q: Wasn't that a little risky?

A: Yeah, they told me I was taking my chances on the temporary, but like I said, I just can't deal with the dentures in the glass. …Sorry.

Q: But it worked out and the bridge held up until second surgery?

A: That's right.

Q: And then these came out when you had your implanted plate put in?

A: Oh yeah, of course they came out.

Q: And you knew they would?

A: Absolutely.

Q: Ok, I'm getting it now. So they removed the four leftovers when they went back to open up the gums to reveal the osseointegrated abutments.

•134• A: You got it.

Q: All right, now just to go over this one time more. To supply a natural foundation for the temporary plate which fits over your gums during the healing process between first and second surgeries, four of your best teeth were left in your mouth.

A: That's right.

Q: Any problems with infection or food getting caught in the bridge?

A: No, I brushed and water-pik'd and everything was fine. They did the first surgery in January, a week later they put in the bridge. Then in the following November they took the bridge out and the four teeth out, then they built the

implant. They build the gums up, they put the healing abutments on, and—it's like construction—they put in this new
mouth. I think by March, I had the permanent upper plate.
But it's like they're custom builders, you know? It's like
every case is done differently, because I guess, every mouth
is different.

Q: Now I don't know how it is for you, but for me, if there's
anything wrong—and I mean anything wrong with my tooth
or gum or cheek—my tongue goes right to it and messes
around 'til it's sore. So every little problem feels huge.
Everything in my mouth is exaggerated. So what I want to
know is what do these teeth feel like, do they feel weird?

•135•

A: No! They feel like mine. I can't get over it. I can't wait 'til
they finish the bottoms, then I'll be the bionic woman. It's
incredible.

Q: And with your significant or insignificant other—as the case
may be—between the two of you… it feels completely natural and comfortable? Mouth-to-mouth resuscitation and the
like?

A: Yeah, it's great. The other, old ones that were glued to the
four remaining teeth—forget about it, I didn't want anyone
near them.

Q: So now you've got the full uppers and you're waiting for the
full lowers.

A: Yeah, we're on stage two for the lowers. They did the first stage surgery again in January, and I went back in March—you know wait six or eight weeks.

Q: Do they always stagger the top and bottom surgeries?

A: I could have done the whole thing at once, but I know about the swelling, and I said no. The bottom swelling goes to the neck, and the top goes up to the eyes. I can wear sunglasses or a scarf, but not both.

Q: So do you smoke cigarettes?

A: Well, I've quit now about three months.

Q: So you quit because...

A: Because I don't want to ruin my new teeth.

Q: So the implants acted as an inspiration?

A: They definitely did. It's a whole new me now.

Q: That's great. Tobacco's a nasty addiction. Some people say it's worse than heroin.

A: Well, thank God I wouldn't know, but it's tough. I thought I would go nuts for a while. Then I got smart, I said, "What's your worse time?" It's in the morning. So I changed my routine, I get up, throw my shorts and a T-shirt on, and do the track. And then I don't have time to linger, I have to get in the shower, get dressed, go to work and start smiling at the world with my new teeth.

Q: Amen. You're a textbook case, all right. And you give a great interview, like they say in Hollywood.

CHAPTER SEVEN

Bone

GRAFTING

Dental implants need a foundation. Bone is that foundation. Osseointegration is the process by which implants are accepted into bone, but implants also require proper bone structure to osseointegrate. If the bony integrity (the volume of bone at the intended implant site) is insufficient, we must replace it before, or simultaneously, to the implant procedure.

Why Does Bone Disappear?

Bone is living tissue and, depending on how it is treated and nourished, it strengthens or weakens. As bone is used it is stimulated and rejuvenates itself, as all healthy living cells do. When bone is not stimulated it shrinks back on itself, a process called "resorbsion." In a healthy mouth, teeth assume hundreds, even thousands of pounds of pressure per square inch. This pressure is passed onto the jawbones, keeping them vital and strong. When teeth are removed for whatever reason, bone is no longer in function, and jawbone begins to resorb. The resorbsion process takes time, but after tooth loss it is inevitable.

If you lose a tooth and come to us for an evaluation within six months of the loss, except in a serious trauma case (wherein bone and/or teeth have been injured), chances are the bone will have suffered very little atrophy and will be of sufficient volume to withstand an implant. On the other hand, if you come to us several years after tooth loss you will have certainly suffered bone atrophy, and you may require bone grafting to increase your bone volume before implants are appropriate.

Bone Augmentation:

We augment bone by filling a defect with some type of material. The most common form of bone augmentation is called "grafting." Dental bone grafting plays an important role in implant scenarios in which structural or functional support is necessary.

Twenty years ago when P. I. Brånemark developed this first truly effective system of dental implants, the procedure proved so taxing to the bone structure, that a considerable number of elderly and/or injured candidates were refused simply because their bone structures were not hearty enough. The only alternative was to subject these patients to involved bone graftings.

Certainly, conventional bone grafting proved effective but added cost, discomfort, and time—as much as six months—to a procedure already testing the tolerances of our quick-fix culture. Traditionally such procedures require that surgeons "harvest" and "re-plant" continuous stretches of strong bone from the patient themselves. "Donor" bone met with some success but also increased the possibility of rejection due to infection or non-compatibility.

Recently, however, breakthroughs in tissue engineering have come to the rescue, and today the percentage of persons we're able to accept as candidates for implants has risen dramatically. The reason being that over the past years researchers have separated bone into its genetic components, isolating the inert "building blocks" to activate bone growth with cells borrowed from elsewhere in the same body.

Mechanisms of Bone Grafting

There are three different processes associated with successful bone grafting:

1) osteogenesis
2) osteoinduction
3) osteoconduction

The first of these, Osteogenesis, is the formation and development of bone in the body. The second, Osteoinduction, is the act or process of stimulating Osteogenesis; and the third, Osteoconduction, provides an armature suitable for repositioning new bone. All grafting materials possess at least one of these modes.

Types of Graft Material

A frequent question of patients is: "Where do you get the bone from?" There are four primary types of bone grafting material: autogenous bone, allografts, alloplasts, and bone substitutes. Autogenous bone: related to dental implant surgery is the transplantation of bone from one region of the body to another (in the same person). This is considered the gold standard of grafting material. Autogenous grafting heals through the processes of osteoinduction, osteoconduction, and osteogenesis. Autogenous bone can be harvested from many sites in the mouth: the back part of the lower jawbone, the chin region, and the back part of the upper jawbone. Other parts of the body often used include: part of the hip bone, part of the lower leg, and part of the skull.

The extra-oral (or non-oral) sites are used most frequently for severe trauma or cancer patients associated with extremely large bone defects and are not commonly used for dental implant grafting. The main disadvantage to such surgeries is that they require two surgeries and two healing sites.

ALLOGRAFT BONE GRAFT:

Bone is obtained from another person through a bone bank or a living donor. Before using a bone bank, speak to your surgeon and make certain the bank is accredited by the American Association of Tissue Banks. An accredited organization (at this time there are only two in the US) deals with a purely non-viable material, which is to say, tissue with no living cells. All bone and tissue is frozen, demineralized, and completely sterilized, without exception. Some of the advantages of allografts include availability and the elimination of the need for the "harvesting" surgery. The disadvantages are primarily associated with the use of tissues from another individual. This type of graft is occasionally rejected by the immune system, as sometimes occurs with other transplanted tissues.

ALLOPLASTS OR SYNTHETIC BONE SUBSTITUTES:

Alloplastic materials are available in a variety of textures, sizes, and shapes. The specific properties of an alloplast determine which synthetic material is best for a particular application. Such bone substitutes include bovine-derived porous bone, synthetic ceramics, and bioactive glass materials.

The most common alloplasts are bovine bone, synthetic calcium phosphate material, and those derived from natural sources, mainly coral. The ceramics operate with an osteoconductive mechanism, which means that such materials are used to reconstruct bony defects by providing a scaffold for enhanced bone repair and growth.

There are a wide array of grafting materials that can be used in a variety of dental applications. Autogenous bone (from the same body) remains the best material because a body never rejects its own bone cells. However, autogenous bone also has some disadvantages, and since it is not needed in every situation, your surgeon will select a specific graft or combination of grafting materials to match a particular dental problem.

INTERVIEW SIX

The patient is a male in his middle 40s who works for a pharmaceutical company in the tri-state area.

Q: Can you tell me a bit about your sinus lift surgery and your implant procedure in general?

A: I can tell you about before and after, the technicalities are something of a blur, and to be truthful—that's how I like it.

Q: That's fine. Fire away.

A: In point of fact, it was my dentist who diagnosed me as a diabetic. Diabetics don't have as rigorous blood circulation as normal people, and that was part of the reason I was losing teeth. Poor circulation means poor capillary action in the gums, less strong bones, less strong teeth, and so forth. It was also part of the reason that I was teetering on the edge of not being able to have implant surgery. In choosing to go forward, I was told we were "pushing the envelope."

• 145 •

Q: Your surgeon told you that going in?

A: He told me, all right. I'm just not so sure I was focusing on what he said.

Q: But there was no other operation on your leg or rib, to harvest bone for grafting?

A: No, just the one surgery, a six-month recuperation period, and then the follow-up.

Q: And how was the recuperation after the sinus lift?

A: Well, that's where the personal attention really does figure in. Because that was the information that did interest me—namely, how much pain and for how long. I'm in the medical education field myself, and I've also had a fair number of surgeries. The thing is that when you feel like you know what's happening and what will happen to you, it greatly diminishes the anxiety surrounding the procedure, and when anxiety diminishes—so does the pain. That's why Valium decreases pain. It's not a painkiller per se, it's an anti-anxiety medication.

Q: So you found the preparation was thorough and effective?

A: That's right. If anything I'd say I was prepared for a bad case scenario, but when I found myself in less pain than I expected I relaxed, and the experience was really rather undramatic. The duration on the other hand did get a bit tedious.

Q: We're speaking of the first surgery, with sinus lift, grafting, and the placement of the abutments.

A: That's right. But let me qualify this...I wouldn't use the word "pain" past the first few days. Well, the first day and a half you don't feel anything. And after that I found the pain bearable.

Q: You were using painkillers by then?

A: Actually, I don't like to use painkillers. Every now and then I'd use some ibuprofen. But after the first week I'd really say the "ache" was gone, and there was simply an unpleasant discomfort. Mild at the gumline and gaining in strength approaching my sinuses. My cheekbones were sensitive, and since this is actually sinus related surgery, my condition was weather-sensitive. On rainy days it was worse than on sunny days.

Q: And so the discomfort lasted how long?

A: Up to five months.

Q: And that discomfort, was it still starting at gumline?

A: No, by then, it was just my sinuses. My cheekbones, actually.

•|47•

Q: And that was from the sinus lift?

A: Right. From that point on it's been smooth sailing, however, the day after tomorrow, I get the final implants placed.

Q: Up to this point you've been using…?

A: A temporary bridge.

Q: Which means you'll have a new full upper plate.

A: And I can start thinking about doing the bottoms.

Q: Is that right?

A: Oh yeah, my new teeth make in clear. After I tried on the final product I knew. Once New Year's rolls around I'll go in for my appointment. I'm very, very happy with my teeth.

Q: And if you don't mind my asking how much the upper set cost?

A: $17,000, and worth every penny. And now I'm late for a meeting so if you have any other questions…

Q: No, that's fine. Thanks so much.

Immediate or "Replace" Implant

• 148 • After all we've told you about two-stage surgeries for the successful implant procedure, there is one modification of this practice. A "replace implant" resembles regular implants in most attributes except that it occurs immediately following the extraction of a tooth.

How it Works

When a tooth is slated for removal from an area that is otherwise healthy, the surgeon prepares the bone socket with some additional drilling, and an "immediate implant" fills the vacuum. This replacement implant relies upon a tapered root-like fixture which duplicates the shape of the missing tooth. Other than this tapered shape a replacement implant is exactly like any other implant, except for the suturing and unsuturing of surrounding gums in the initial two weeks accompanying normal first stage surgery. Other than that the careful regime surrounding the osseointegration process remains the same.

The advantage of immediate implant placement lies in saving time—finished teeth a week or two sooner. Again the surgeon will judge if you are a candidate for immediate implant placement. Specific criteria apply.

INTERVIEW SEVEN

Subject is an accountant living in New York City.

Q: Could you tell me about how you came to dental implants?

A: Sure. About 15 years ago my dentist told me I had gum disease and recommended a periodontist, who treated me. But still the teeth in the back of my mouth continued to get dark, and while I was eating a lamb chop, I lost one. And that was the beginning of a nightmare—one after another I began losing teeth.

Q: So they tried to save your original teeth and failed?

A: Right. Over the years I had them scraped, and that seemed to work for a while, but eventually the roots weakened, the teeth darkened, and fell out.

Q: Did you have false teeth put in?

A: No, it was in the back, so I just chewed more in the front sections of my mouth.

Q: But always worrying about the next disaster, having to be careful of everything you bite—it's a private little agony if nothing else?

A: That's right. And then I heard about implants. I'd known about them for quite a while, and I knew they would cost a fair amount of money, but I didn't want dentures and I decided that I would go for the implants. Of course I didn't know exactly what would be involved, but I decided that implants were the only realistic option.

Q: So you could afford the implants, and you felt you had the psychological make-up to go through the ordeal of the two surgeries, etc?

A: Well, I didn't know it would be quite as involved as it turned out to be.

Q: Ok, here's a tricky question. You say you didn't know it would be as involved a procedure. Now is that because you didn't want to hear it, or didn't understand it, or because it wasn't properly explained?

A: It wasn't fully communicated, I don't think. I mean they tell you, but they can't really tell you.

Q: Well, if somehow they could have told you—would it have changed your mind?

A: No.

Q: So in a sense you're glad that you didn't know.

A: That's right.

Q: So what exactly was the process for you, did you do tops and bottoms both?

A: No, I'm doing the tops. And I don't need to do the bottoms yet, maybe in ten years, but not for now.

•|5|•

Q: Were you a typical case or—

A: Well, I had eight implants put in my upper jaw. All in one sitting. They said they'd never done so many in an upper jaw. I did lose two out of the eight, and they did bone grafting on the second surgery and placed the two back in.

Q: In the same surgery?

A: Yeah, it was the second surgery for the other six, and they put replacement implants in for the other two.

Q: So are you wearing temporary dentures at the moment?

A: No, they've cemented a plate onto the healthy implants which holds really well, actually, even though it will hold even better once all eight posts are fully healed. One side of my mouth has all four and the other side has only two fully healed, so they'll go back in and reopen the two new implants and build them up, and then I'll be done.

Q: So how many pieces in your final prosthesis?

A: There are two, dividing at the front teeth.

Q: And when was your first operation?

A: May of '98.

Q: So that's 16 months ago. And you'll be done when?

A: January or February.

Q: Which will make it a total of 24 months, give or take a few weeks. And do you mind my asking you what the final cost will be?

A: The final cost will be $24,000, not including gas, tolls, and parking in Manhattan. And I'm incredibly happy with the whole thing.

Q: Are you married or single?

A: I'm single.

Q: So do you feel a little more confident in your social life?

A: Yeah. People told me, from the moment I had the plate put in, that I started to smile with my teeth exposed. I didn't realize that I'd been keeping my mouth shut to try and cover my teeth, and that changed—well, they said it changed from one day to the next.

Q: That's great. And one relaxes from that point on, I think one's whole manner is looser and happier.

A: That's right. As I said before, I'm very happy with my implants.

Q: Well, congratulations and thanks for talking with me.

•153•

CHAPTER EIGHT

MAINTENANCE

You don't often see a new Mercedes covered with mud. The reason being that when a person takes trouble enough to equip themselves with a beautiful, expensive automobile they usually protect their investment and take a measure of pride in owning "the best."

In the case of dental implants we take this pride and protectiveness a step further. For an implant is not merely a possession, it is an adopted part of you. You've worked hard to rehabilitate your smile, your laugh, your ability to eat and socialize without anxiety or pain.

Your implants—we have every reason to believe—will change your life so much, we'd start sounding like Hallmark card writers were we to really list the thousand and one ways your life will be improved. But here's the hook. You have to clean your implants. Every day. If you do you'll prevent your gums from retracting, prevent bone loss beneath the gums, and help guarantee that osseointegration will remain "rock-hard" for the rest of your life.

Saliva is nature's tooth cleaner. During sleep you don't secrete as much saliva, so that even when you haven't eaten a thing, bacteria has a nice long incubation period to create "morning breath." Those of you with implants will want to eliminate that first batch of bacteria, first thing in the day, and last thing at night. At any rate, this is the ideal scenario. If, for some reason, you have time later in the day to really do a fine job of cleaning your new teeth, this is fine. But everyday!

Some of you may be thinking, "Where is all your talk of 'bionic this,' and 'indestructible that' if I have to clean these superhuman chompers as vigilantly or MORE than regular ol' teeth?"

One answer is: vanity. Who would buy a Mercedes and then leave it dirty and unpolished? Shine those implants up—and let them do their job as ambassadors of brightness. The other answer is: prevention of bone loss. And the third is: infection. Yes, your implants are totally resistant to conventional decay. But because they are indeed artificial, because they don't consist of nerve and bone connected to your bloodstream, they are honored "guests" in your mouth. And like guests, as opposed to family, they require a little more attention.

•157•

The most high-maintenance implant is the permanent full bridge—upper or lower—doesn't matter. Food gets lodged between gums and prosthesis, this becomes both uncomfortable and—if left for more than ten hours—unhealthy. Haven't you spent enough time in the dental chair? Do you really want more problems when you could be trouble free? With daily cleaning we safeguard against infection and keep our office check-ups to a minimum. Dental hygienists use special instruments to clean around the abutments four times a year. So let's get down to your own cleaning procedures at home dealing with the most demanding cases first. First thing: put together a bag of cleaning articles that you can pick up and take with you in your new, socially demanding life.

Your cleaning kit should include:

(1) flossing yarn

(2) crochet hook

(3) small-end tufted (soft) toothbrush

(4) interproximal brush

(5) toothpaste

(6) reading glasses

FIRST: To clean the abutment posts (which stick through the gums onto which your bridge is attached), loop cotton ribbon or thick floss around the rear of the post and back out through the front. It helps to use a crochet hook to seize the ribbon and drag it free. Coat a section of ribbon with toothpaste and pull this back forth as a rag shines a shoe. You may find it efficient to snake your floss in a sideways "S" around three posts and then perform the back-and-forth motion.

The single-tuft brush is used to clean the abutment buccally and lingually (tongue side and cheek side).

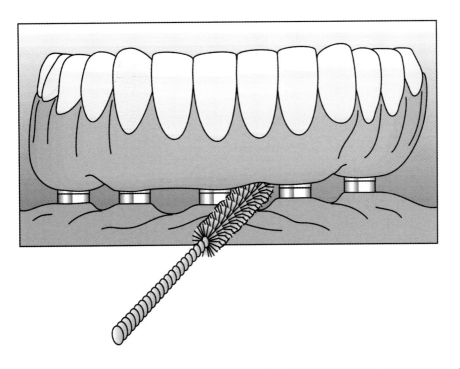

The interdental brush is used between the abutments and the base of the denture and gums.

NEXT: (in either of the aforementioned techniques) slacken your ribbon between a given set of posts and grab some excess. If you are working on the bottom arch pull up, if the top arch, pull down. Now perform the same back-and-forth action shifting the "scrub" from the lateral cleaning of the posts, to an up-and-down cleaning of the underside of the prosthesis.

Many find the additional use of an interproximal brush massages the gums and helps to clean the underside of the prosthesis and the abutment posts. This device can be used at a restaurant or at the office, more quickly and casually. Add a dab of toothpaste for an even better clean.

If you need hands-on instruction the dentist or hygienist will provide a demonstration.

To clean the teeth themselves (this applies to a bridge, partial bridge, or single-tooth implants), create a pattern and stick to it.

For instance (in the case of a full arch): With your toothpaste and soft toothbrush begin on the left back teeth.

(1) Brush the backs and tops as you would conventional teeth.

(2) Proceed to midsection (front) teeth, brushing the backs and whichever sections of the abutments posts can be reached.

(3) Now brush the right rear teeth as you did the left.

(4) Swing back to the left side and brush back teeth's outer surfaces.

(5) Come center and brush the outer front teeth and whichever sections of abutment posts can be reached.

(6) Finish with the back teeth of the right side, brushing the outer surfaces.

(7) Now take your brush and attend to the very bottom edge of the prosthesis, closest to the gum. Rinse thoroughly, some prefer to used a Water-Pik, although this device cannot be substituted for the manual cleaning just outlined.

(8) SMILE!

Removable Teeth:

Clean the prosthesis in place, first, as outlined in the previous paragraph. Then remove the bridge, clean the bare abutments with the ribbon as first explained, then, holding the prosthesis upside down, tend to the bottom of the bridge with toothpaste on a rag.

Gentle pressure will do. Rinse thoroughly and replace.

Remember: Most of this is a new ritual, like learning to tie your first shoelace. Few of these procedures will be "natural" the first time. Allow yourself to be less-than-perfect at all of this.

•161•

CHAPTER NINE

Are Implants for ME?

A Cynic's Conversion

In the last analysis, explaining every technique of dental implantology isn't practical, because implantology is a technical science which borders on the realm of art. When a millionaire hires a captain to skipper his yacht and rough weather sets in, the wealthy customer is probably below deck, unaware of the rules that are bent or even broken as the veteran seaman plies his lifesaving skills. What matters is that the ship is whole and everyone is smiling when the sun comes out. What matters is that "it all comes out fine in the end." In a sense, you must place that same sort of trust in the hands of your dental implantology team. Which doesn't mean you shouldn't question long and hard before that final leap of faith.

INTERVIEW EIGHT

We illustrate the point with an interview with one of our favorite patients, a Holocaust survivor, who spoke with a research assistant in November of '98.

Q: You had your implants put in how long ago, ma'am?

A: Seven, eight years.

Q: Can you describe to me what brought you to make this decision?

A: We knew Dr. Wiland for a long time. I started with good teeth, but you get older and it all changes. So he kept telling me here and there, these teeth are loose, but I resisted. Until

I couldn't even bite into a piece of soft bread. It was so painful, but I kept on telling him, "Please, Doctor Wiland you have to make me a denture." And he'd insist, "But you don't have the gums for dentures! If I make you dentures it's I who will suffer because you'll cry on my shoulder." Then he'd put his hand on my hand and say, "You have to have implants!" Until I finally told him that if he told me about implants one more time that I, along with my entire family, would stop going to him as our dentist. Because, you know, I used to read about implants, a lot of bad stories.

Q: The blade implants?

A: Right. We knew somebody who was more in the hospital than she was at home after she had those put in.

Q: Dr. Wiland experimented with them years ago, but then decided they didn't work and stopped using them.

A: Yeah, sure. They've come such a long way with such a lot things like the heart and the hip and knee—whatever you need, almost, they can make a surgery for...I mean, thank God they can patch us up.

Q: So when did you finally give in to Dr. Wiland's request?

A: He finally came to me and said, "Please listen to me, we have a video I would like you and your husband to watch." I said, "Don't you dare give me a video..." But finally, I couldn't take it anymore, I couldn't eat, I had lost weight, you know. I had the caps but they were loose.

Then he told me a story about his mother-in-law.

Now we all know what you guys think of your mothers-in-law, but she was in so much pain that even the cold heart of a son-in-law was touched, so he made an implant for her and now they get along near perfect because it worked out so well. So God should only bless him—because he told me that story, and I finally listened. And now there is not a thing I can't eat. Old fashioned bread with a crust, an apple...I haven't bitten into an apple for 20 years! And now, after Thanksgiving, I'm ready to go to have them taken out and cleaned.

Q: Good. You go every year?

A: I don't go every year, because I do a good job for myself. I rinse with soda water twice a day, and I massage my gums. *(Laughs)*

Q: Now tell me, you had the implants placed in the lower jaw and it took—what— four or five months to heal?

A: Well, you know, one thing—they cut and make surgery...

Q: You were conscious?

A: Oh, yes. Yes it took five months to heal.

Q: I believe you had six implants put in.

A: Yes—five or six—I didn't lose any. I know. Every one took and they all work fine today. You know, Dr. Wiland knocks on them when I have them cleaned, and he tells they are good—perfect.

Q: Then after they put in the implants, they installed a temporary bridge.

A: Yeah—I don't wish it on my enemy.

•167•

Q: The temporary, you mean?

A: When I was in the house, I kept them in the drawer.

Q: They were painful to wear?

A: Yes, very painful. I didn't have the gums—you see—nothing to rest on. But all that's over now.

Q: After the unfortunate part with the temporaries, they went back in and they put the teeth on...

A: Yes.

Q: Was there still some pain with that part of the process?

A: Nothing. Just little adjustments. Nothing serious, no pain.

Q: Did it interfere with your speech at all?

A: Not at all.

Q: And do you feel comfortable smiling?

A: Are you kidding? I have the nicest smile on the block! *(Quietly)* And I want you to know, people think it's caps. Dr. Wiland did a great job...you see, it's very important when they put on the teeth—the implants are fine—but the teeth—are very important, you know...how they look when he puts on the teeth. Yes, yes. The whole thing took a year and a half, two years, and I'm grateful that finally he convinced me. Dr. Wiland is a wonderful man—like family.

Q: You mind if I ask your age, ma'am.

A: I'm 70.

Q: So you had this done when you were 62?

A: That's right, thank God he convinced me.

Q: And would you mind if I asked you how much the whole thing cost?

A: The whole thing? Was almost $12,000. Worth every penny.

Of course, today it's more again. But the worse part—

Q: What was the worst part?

A: After he finally convinced me that there was nothing else he could do for me, that I had no choice but to do the implants, then he says: "And now you have to do tests to see if you're a candidate." After all that! What? They were going to tell me no, I couldn't do it? *(Laughs)* But I passed the tests and on we went—thank God!"

•169•

AFTERWORD

We have tried to outline, illustrate, and simplify the various aspects of implant dentistry with all of its possible applications for you.

All of these procedures are currently available and are the accepted standard of care. Every year hundreds of thousands of dental implant cases are completed successfully. So successfully that the procedure "works" more than 94% of the time, a statistic that is more successful than most medical procedures. We have answered many questions in this book, such as, "Do I have enough bone?" The answer usually has been yes. Sometimes "yes" with a surgeon's help with bone grafting. Now we are routinely using the patient's Protein Rich Plasma (PRP) and the growth factors within to jump start the integration of bone grafts and the growth of his or her own bone.

Genetics Institute has isolated and is producing Bone Morphogenic Protein (BMP) in the form of a clear liquid that when placed in an area where we want bone to grow will make it grow. In many cases that will help us to restore form to the jaws, and with the help of osseointegrated dental implants restore function—the ability to chew and enjoy food.

The bio-mechanics of dental implants are well known in almost all their biological applications, and research is being done the world over to make them even better. But there still are some areas that we need to focus on specifically, and other areas where breakthroughs have occurred that need to be brought forth.

Two procedures, both of which require specific training, are placing and restoring of the zygomaticus fixture. The procedure has applications in special situations in which a patient has no bone covering the sinus and cannot have a bone graft. There are many patients who, because of trauma, cancer, or disease, can be helped with this proven restorative option.

Nobel Biocare has introduced a dental implant procedure called Novum Protocol for same-day teeth. This protocol, which is executed by a team consisting of an oral surgeon, a restorative dentist, and a laboratory technician, can provide a stable bone-anchored bridge in eight hours. The success rate for fixed bridge stability in the mandible is in the range of 95% to 100% in more than 10 years of function, according to pre-introduction studies done in many parts of the world.

There are some problems which have not been solved yet, but we are working very hard to give acceptable aesthetic results. These problems don't involve case longevity or stability or functionality or even the smile, they involve the way teeth on implants come out of the gums or, in dentist language, the emergence profile of the new bionic restorations. Thanks to the periodontists, they are getting better and with bone grafting advances, teeth are not made as long as they were previously.

As clinicians, we have seen a greater advance in dentistry in the last 40 years than in the last 4000 years; and at the present rate of advancement, the next 10 years will hopefully give us what we would like: faster osseointegration, faster integration of bone grafting, and soft tissue engineering that will give us the ability to shape the gums and supporting tissues like a plastic surgeon does in a facelift. This is not only possible, but probable in the near future.

We have come a long way from full dentures that have been in a glass of water throughout the night, being placed on sore gums in the morning. We have come a long way from partial dentures that clasp abutment teeth and eventually loosen the teeth to which they are attached. We have come a long way from cutting down virgin teeth to replace a missing tooth. We have come a long way in giving cancer and trauma victims functioning and aesthetically pleasing mouths and smiles.

If you need us, the dental profession is at your service.

SMILE

SMILE